Praise for Dr. Cunningham and His Book

Dr. Cunningham has achieved two remarkable feats: First, he and his group are unique in undertaking and intelligently interpreting the results of a comprehensive, rigorous, and prospective study of qualities that favor cancer survival. Secondly, he has written the clearest, most balanced, and objectively critical perspective on several decades of research into the question of whether and how the mind can affect health and disease, particularly cancer. The glow from Dr. Cunningham's accumulated experience and wisdom literally illuminates the field, and indicates a pathway to healing for those living with cancer.
   —LYDIA R. TEMOSHOK, PhD
      Professor of Medicine and Psychiatry
      University of Maryland School of Medicine, Baltimore

This is the most thoughtful discussion of what makes group support most effective and supportive. Every oncology professional should read this book.
   —JAMES S. GORDON, MD
      Founder and director of the Center for Mind-Body Medicine,
      clinical professor in the Departments of Psychiatry and Family
      Medicine at the Georgetown University School of Medicine,
      author of *Comprehensive Cancer Care: Integrating Alternative,
      Complementary and Conventional Therapies*, and *Manifesto for a
      New Medicine: Your Guide to Healing Partnerships and the Wise Use of
      Alternative Therapies*

D0981479

This book clearly and systematically brings together a comprehensive picture of current holistic thinking, research and findings in the field . . . it is readily comprehensible by both new and experienced practitioners as well as by lay people.

—RUTH BOLLETINO, PhD

Psychotherapist in New York City specializing in work with people with cancer and other life-threatening illnesses

Carefully making the case that the mind, under certain conditions, can beneficially alter the course of cancer, Alastair Cunningham—who has worked with cancer patients and studied the results for many years—takes on an enormously important issue that most members of the medical profession do not consider worth examining. His thoughtful, non-contentious, and eminently sensible book, a signal effort to integrate a variety of findings and assessments within a single framework, will inform researchers, practitioners, and patients.

—HARRIS DIENSTFREY

Editor of *Advances in Mind-Body Medicine*, 1991–2001, author of *Where the Mind Meets the Body*

Can the Mind Heal Cancer?

A Clinician-Scientist Examines the Evidence

ALASTAIR J. CUNNINGHAM

OC, PhD, C.Psych.

2005

Other books by the author
Understanding Immunology (1978)
The Healing Journey (1992, 2000)
Bringing Spirituality into Your Healing Journey (2002)

Library and Archives Canada Cataloguing in Publication

Cunningham, Alastair J. (Alastair James), 1940–
Can the mind heal cancer? : a clinician-scientist examines the evidence /
Alastair J. Cunningham.
ISBN 0-9737854-0-3
1. Cancer—Psychological aspects. 2. Mind and body. 1. Title.
RC262.C84 2005   616.994'0019   C2005-903465-3

Cover illustration: "Through my psychological and spiritual work I feel that I am opening up so that the light in me can merge with the light all around." The artist was a woman with cancer of the pancreas who outlived her prognosis by 2 years.

Table of Contents

Illustrations

Preface

This short book is a presentation of the case that people with cancer, or other serious diseases, who use psychological and spiritual methods in the struggle to heal—who in other words, use their minds—are likely to live much longer than medically predicted. That is the conclusion I have come to after some 40 years in cancer-related research and clinical practice. Our medical system is admirable in many respects, but there is a vital element missing from it: the mind of the person with the disease. Healing can be much more effective if the patient's mind becomes involved. It is a potential that we probably all possess but that few invoke. Our society, and in particular our health care system, does not endorse it yet. Most critics have not studied the evidence, and it is not readily available in one place. I have tried to draw the strands together here.

My own exposure to cancer research began in the 1960s, at the Australian National University, where I was a researcher in the field of immunology. At that time, there were high hopes that this discipline was going to provide an eventual cure for many cancers. By the time I moved to the Ontario Cancer Institute in Toronto, Canada, in 1977, this goal was no closer to realization, and in fact, many of us could see that it probably would not happen. As a result I began questioning my own motives and could not avoid the conclusion that the research I was doing, while interesting in itself, was unlikely to help any of the cancer patients who surrounded us in the hospital where I was now located. A period of transition followed, made possible by the tolerance and support of my superiors, after which I ended up with a second PhD, in clinical psychology this time, and with a new line of work—conducting group classes and therapy for cancer patients, and evaluating their effect. This is the work I've been engaged in for the last 23 years. During that time I've had the opportunity to observe thousands of people with cancer who have come to our program wanting help to cope with their disease and to improve their chances of survival, where possible. Together with a small team of assistants, I have carried out a lot of research on the way peoples' quality of life almost always improves, sometimes dramatically, through learning relatively simple coping skills like deep relaxation, mental imaging, meditation, and thought management.

More recently we have also examined the effect of self-help work of this kind on the lifespan in people with medically incurable cancers. The heart of this book is a series of studies, conducted over the last 10 years, on the mental qualities that people with medically incurable cancers develop during their struggle with the disease. Some individuals become very involved in helping themselves through psychological and spiritual growth or change, and this is often (not always) associated with surviving much longer than predicted by their oncologists. Others do not become involved in this way, and tend to die in about the time predicted by experts. Those who do greatly outlive their prognoses tend to show a pattern of qualities that is also described in reports over the last few decades on studies of "remarkable survivors": these qualities include *autonomy*, or achieving a sense of free choice to live life as desired, the related property of *authenticity*, or learning one's true identity through introspective psychological and spiritual work, and *acceptance*, an attitude of tolerance, forgiveness, and ultimately love for other people, themselves, and all living things. In fact, we scientists, struggling naively to document healing change, appear to have rediscovered a "healed" state of mind that is described in the major wisdom traditions of humankind. It is perhaps not surprising that such a healed mental state promotes physical healing.

While the convergence of evidence on the mental correlates of bodily healing is reassuring, there is another line of evidence that allows us to anchor these findings in a simple, non-technical, and quite conservative theory. This is the pioneering work of U.S. researcher

Lydia Temoshok who, with Henry Dreher, described a "Type C" personality in people susceptible to certain types of cancer. It was found that poorer outcomes were associated with an attitude of "niceness," emotional suppression, and eagerness to placate while denying one's own legitimate needs. This is virtually a mirror image of the authentic, autonomous way of life that we, and others, have seen long survivors develop. The theory then becomes, in outline: if we place undue stress or strain upon ourselves from an early age, we will be susceptible to later disease (Temoshok proposed this theory for cancer, and it may be true for many chronic diseases, different kinds of distortion predisposing us to different conditions). And conversely, if we strive to undo these distortions, to reclaim our authentic selves when afflicted by cancer, we allow our innate healing mechanisms the best opportunity to overcome, or at least retard, the disease.

The evidence behind this simple view will need to be reproduced many times by many scientists before it is generally accepted. This will take decades. Meanwhile, people are suffering more than is necessary. We can say quite definitely that when people with cancer become involved in helping themselves psychologically and spiritually, they almost always enjoy a much better quality of life. It is highly probable, if not yet proven to the satisfaction of all, that some will live much longer as a result.

A further, important experience has shaped my opinions on all of this. In 1987 I had a serious (Stage III) colon cancer myself. Surgery and chemotherapy followed, but I also tried to practise what at that time I was already preaching, and took myself off to a retreat centre for 3 months where, with a group of people learning to be yoga teachers, I spent 10 hours a day, 7 days a week working on my own psychological and spiritual growth. I was strongly motivated because my prognosis was only "one chance in three of long-term survival." Through the personal work I confirmed for myself, in a way that no academic study could do, the truth of what the mystics have expounded on the authentic self. I also had a number of unusual, "paranormal" experiences around that time. My spiritual (not religious) study intensified, and has remained central for me to this day. It has spilled over into our work at the hospital, of course; I now feel that counselling people who have life-threatening disease without addressing the spiritual dimension (where they are open to it) is rather like trying to do marital counselling without talking about sex!

The sum of these experiences—laboratory and clinical research and practice, the psychological counselling, the insights that my own cancer and spiritual work have provided—supply the motivation for writing this book. It's an unusually broad background that has given me sympathy for both the clinician and the researcher, for the intuitive layperson, and for the professional. All have a contribution to make. We need, however, to balance the enthusiasm of the intuitive lay healer, who may want to claim that anyone can heal himself using simple psychological strategies, against the cautious conservatism of the objective professional, who sees the biases in many of the New Age claims. We must take into account the practical difficulties that the working clinician encounters in helping the ordinary person get in touch with his own emotional and spiritual potential. Nevertheless, the possibility of assisting people much more profoundly than we usually do is very clear to me now, as it is to a number of other clinicians and scientists in the health field.

The book is not written as a technical treatise, but is meant to be accessible both to thoughtful lay persons and to health care professionals. I have tried to "digest" the concepts and present them in palatable form. It is not primarily a self-help book for cancer patients—I have published two other books of this kind, listed in references to chapter 1—but a review of ideas and evidence underlying a rational self-help approach. Nor is it an anthology of stories about individuals triumphing over disease; these can be inspiring for people with a serious disease, but there are already many such books on the market.

Beyond the specifics of opposing cancer I am also suggesting new ways of looking at the mind–body relationship and healing. What is true for cancer will doubtless be true for many other serious chronic diseases. And what we may learn from our efforts to heal disease may teach us a great deal about healing all aspects of our lives.

The Ontario Cancer Institute in Toronto has for many years provided a supportive environment for our efforts to learn more about how to help people with cancer through psychological and spiritual work and change. Colleagues who have been particularly involved in the research, or in organizing our group therapy programs have included Dr. Claire Edmonds, Dr. Cathy Phillips, Dr. David Hedley, Ms. Kim Watson, Ms. Gina Lockwood, Ms. Jan Ferguson, Ms. Krista Soots, Dr. Joanne Stephen, Mr. Hayman Buwaneswaran and Ms. Amy Lee. Dr. Edmonds and Ms. Watson assisted with preparation of the chapter references, and they and Drs. Phillips and Hedley read part or all of the manuscript. Mr. Ian MacKenzie kindly prepared the manuscript for publication.

My gratitude and respect extend to the many thousands of patients who have participated in our classes over the years, and especially to those individuals who have courageously persisted with their self-healing work, and in doing so taught us what the human mind and spirit can do. As always, I am deeply grateful to my wife Margaret, for helping with many of our advanced groups and for her unwavering love and support.

—Alastair Cunningham, March 2005

Chapter 1

Can the Mind Heal Cancer?
Popular and Professional Views

INTRODUCTION

Can the mind heal cancer? This is a question that often comes up in the popular press: we read stories of people who seem to have overcome their disease, and these stories provide encouragement to some of the many thousands who are struggling with cancer themselves. Yet health professionals shake their heads in dismay at the popularization of this notion that the mind might affect the way cancer progresses: it seems highly improbable to most of them that an intangible thing like "mind" could significantly influence a concrete, organic disease like cancer.

I am caught somewhere in the middle of this debate. As a health psychologist, scientist. and cancer survivor, I have been professionally engaged in cancer research for 40 years, first as an immunologist, then for the last 25 years from the point of view of a psychologist studying the healing potential of mind. I have watched several thousand people with cancer attempt to alleviate their suffering and influence their disease through deliberate mental action, and I've worked in this way with my own disease. My team and I are one of a small number of groups around the world who are doing systematic research on this question. We belong to a new field, a branch of health psychology, called "psycho-oncology," which is concerned with both the impact of cancer on people's minds and with the reverse, the influence of psychological states on the suffering cancer causes and on the disease itself. As a result of our research and that of others, I believe it is now possible to make a plausible case, based on evidence, that certain kinds of mental change may oppose the progression of at least some cancers. This book makes that case, in largely non-technical language so as to be accessible to both laypersons and professionals.

After a general introduction to the topic of mind-assisted healing of cancer in this chapter, I discuss, in chapter 2, how the impact of mind on body may be understood in simple terms, and will offer examples from medicine and health psychology. In chapter 3, we will briefly review some fairly old research on "remarkable survivors," people with cancer who seem to have greatly outlived their expected survival time. There are flaws in this research that are very obvious to health professionals, as will be acknowledged. In chapter 4 I review recent attempts to see whether psychological therapy can extend life in cancer patients. The results of these experiments have been disappointing, but I argue that this is because the methods used have not been suited to detecting prolonged survival in a minority of exceptional patients. Then in chapters 5 and 6 I provide a fairly detailed description of our own recent research in this area, using methods that are able to detect the exceptional patients who make significant efforts to affect the outcome of their disease. We have demonstrated a clear relationship between what we call "involvement in self-help" and significantly longer survival from advanced cancers. This new evidence fits well with the older studies on "remarkable survivors," flawed though these early studies may be, and with certain earlier work on the relationship between coping style and cancer susceptibility. The result of this synthesis is a simple, practical, and evidence-based view of what people can do themselves to aid their healing. I end, in chapter 7, with an attempt to show that healing at the spiritual level may be understood in much the same way as "mind–body" healing, but at a more profound level, namely as the recovery of an authentic sense of self.

WHAT IS HEALING?

"Can the mind heal cancer?" is a very broad question, with a range of possible meanings. The questioner might intend to ask, "Is there some simple mental trick that will reverse and remove a cancer?" Or she might mean, "If I change my behaviours (which begin in the mind), and get my life in order—for example, by changing my diet, doing more exercise, and working less—will that cure my cancer?" Another possible meaning is, "Did my 'personality,' or my attitudes to life, cause my cancer, and if so, can I heal by changing them?" We need first to define what we mean by "healing" before we can approach these questions. This step is all the more necessary because there is so much misunderstanding around the whole subject of mind–body healing, a confusion that contributes to the strong emotions and polarization of opinions, as we shall see.

"Healing" has many facets. The medical view is perhaps the dominant one: *Dorland's Medical Dictionary* (13th edition) describes healing as "the restoration of wounded parts," the focus being mainly on the physical body. The *Oxford English Dictionary* offers a broader definition: "to make whole or sound, to cure (a disease or wound), and also to save, purify, cleanse, repair, amend." Thus although healing involves the restoration of physical health, it can be given a broader meaning, "amending" or putting things to rights. It implies the restoration of harmony, balance, and optimal functioning at all levels of a person (we will expand on this point shortly). There is obviously room for some difference in opinion as to what might be "optimal," but I think most of us would agree on what a healed state would feel like.

Healing can be divided into two broad categories, which we may call "spontaneous" and "assisted." The first is what the body does by itself, without any deliberate intervention by the owner of the body, or by others. There are many spontaneous or automatic healing mechanisms operating constantly in the body and mind; for example, healing of wounds, the immune response to foreign micro-organisms, or, at the mental level, the lessening of anxiety or depression with the passage of time. Assisted healing, by contrast, denotes some kind of active intervention, by the person herself, or by others.

Assisted healing can usefully be divided into two further categories (as shown in Table 1.1). The first is healing promoted by interventions from outside the individual, such as the introduction of foreign materials (food, drugs) to the body. The second is healing caused by changes initiated within the person, which means, essentially, by changes in thoughts and emotional reactions. Some examples may clarify this distinction between externally and internally assisted healing. The former grouping covers almost all standard Western medical practices, and also much of what is called "alternative" medicine, that is, the administration of drugs or procedures by an external person, or by the individual herself. This would include diets or additives used as treatments. Internally assisted healing, by contrast, involves the deliberate invoking, by the individual, of the potentials of his or her own mind and spirit, to facilitate a restoring of harmony and good functioning. We could also call this "mind-mediated," "mind–body," "self-directed" healing, or "self-healing" for short.

Assisted healing can involve both external and internal routes or processes at the same time. Changing behaviours obviously includes both kinds. For example, if someone goes to a dietitian for advice, then adopts a new and healthier diet, he is obviously receiving external assistance and using externally applied agents (food), but much of his healing depends on the internal resolve to monitor the mind's cravings and control them. Another example of overlap would be the help supplied by a psychotherapist (external), leading to inner change by the client (internal).

This distinction between external and internal is a critical one. Externally assisted healing entails looking to some other person or some external agent for relief. Internally assisted healing is what is

4

TABLE 1.1   *Different Routes to Healing*

Spontaneous Healing: What the body and mind can do without any deliberate intervention by anyone, e.g., healing of wounds, immune responses, the lessening of suffering over time.

Assisted Healing: Healing aided by active intervention

1. *Externally Assisted*: Agents or procedures are applied to the sufferer from outside, either by oneself or by others (e.g., drugs, surgery, healthy behaviours like exercise and good diet)

2. *Internally Assisted*: The individual sufferer makes voluntary mental changes to try to affect the health of the body or mind.

Note that 1 and 2 can overlap; thus, adopting a special diet involves introducing external agents (foods), but there is also a large component of voluntary mental change required, which is internal.

normally meant when people speak of "healing through the mind" or "self-healing": it implies a looking within, at one's own attitudes, beliefs, and experiences. The emphasis in self-healing is on changing states of mind rather than simple behavioural change or on manipulating external circumstances. Various techniques (described in two earlier books)[1] are used in healing through the mind: monitoring and controlling one's thoughts, relaxation, mental imagery, meditation, goal setting, as well as techniques from various schools of psychotherapy and spiritual traditions. It is healing by the internal route that is the subject of this book.

THE "LEVELS" OF A PERSON

I want now to introduce a simple diagram (Figure 1.1) that we have found very useful in our work with cancer patients. The five circles of

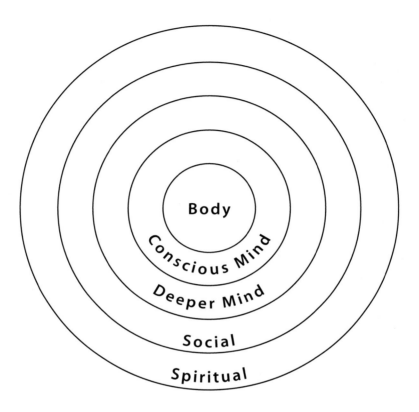

FIGURE 1.1 *A simple "map" showing major levels or dimensions of the human being*

the diagram represent five major human functions or levels: the body, which is our material substrate, or "hardware"; the conscious mind, meaning the stream of thoughts; the deeper mind, a non-technical term intended to lump together our emotions, images, dreams, and impulses operating outside of our awareness; the social level, that part of us that connects in a vital web of relationships to other people; and a spiritual dimension, meaning our connection to a non-material, transcendent substrate or Divine Ground (discussed further in chapter 7). This subdivision can help us understand the variety of events often referred to under the heading of "healing." At the level of the body, it is clear enough: healing means restoring normal balance and function, or what is often called "cure." Healing of the mind means, likewise, that mental functioning is brought back to normal, suffering being relieved. When we talk about healing of suffering, we are, as a moment's reflection will show, really speaking of changes in the mind rather than the body. The suffering caused by cancer, or other serious disease, comes from our horrified reaction to the diagnosis and its implications, and to any unwanted changes that take place in the body. Even pain, although the sensations may arise in the body, is ultimately a mental phenomenon. Healing of our emotional and social levels are likewise intimately connected to whatever is happening in the mind. Healing at the spiritual level is less obvious, and discussion of it will be pursued later; we can say, for the present, that it entails making a strong connection with a transcendent or spiritual order.

The levels in Figure 1.1 are not, of course, really separate; each affects all of the others. A physical change may alter one's thinking and emotions profoundly. Similarly, a change originating in the mind, such as anxiety, may dramatically alter behaviours and ultimately general health status. The mind, as will be seen, tends to be the key level: suffering occurs there, as do the positive experiences of joy, peace, and love. The satisfaction we get from social interactions depends on how we construe them with our minds. The state of mind radiates, as it were, to all other levels. When we refer to healing *through* the mind, we mean that some other part of the individual, usually the body, is being returned to a healthier state by an action of the mind. Likewise healing through the spirit—an unconventional, not to say esoteric idea—would apply if it was thought that some non-material spiritual agency acted upon a person.

I hope this is clear. The definitions are necessary so that we know just what kinds of phenomena we are referring to when we discuss healing. While the principal topic of this book is healing of the body through the mind (internally assisted healing), we will also be concerned with the healing or relief of mental suffering, which is of at least equal importance, and is particularly amenable to change by voluntary mental action on the part of the affected person.

REPHRASING THE QUESTION: "CAN THE MIND HEAL CANCER?"

Let us now examine, in a more precise way, some of the questions that are often asked about what the people can do with their minds to assist themselves in the struggle with cancer:

1. The first might be, "Can the suffering that cancer brings be lessened by voluntary mental action?" The answer to this question is an emphatic yes. Many professionals have concluded that people in such dire trouble can be taught simple methods to help themselves substantially (and we will see that the same holds true for other conditions, like chronic pain), although such education is not usually a part of regular health care.

2. A second question, "Can our behaviours (which originate in our minds) affect the onset of cancer, or the course of an existing cancer?" We can say yes to the first part of this question: an extensive range of scientific literature shows that the risk of getting cancer can be reduced by as much as two-thirds to three-quarters by adopting healthy habits, such as avoiding smoking, eating a healthy diet, and making other lifestyle adjustments (avoiding sunburn, using appropriate protection during sexual contact, avoiding industrial cancer-producing agents). Many things are already being done at a societal level about this; much more is obviously possible (making tobacco an illegal drug, for example). To the second part of this question—do such behaviours affect *existing* cancers—we would have to say that there is no conclusive evidence or consensus among experts yet that simple behav-

ioural change affects cancer progression, beyond affecting general health. This in spite of the fact that many people with cancer attach great hopes to diet, in particular.

3.   A third question is much more controversial: "Can we use our minds to beneficially affect the course of an existing cancer?" In other words, is internally assisted healing of physical cancer possible, through the agency of mind? This is what people usually mean when they ask, "Can the mind heal cancer?" It is perhaps the most intellectually fascinating and emotionally compelling issue in the modern research field of "psycho-oncology," which deals with all aspects of the relationship between cancer and the mind, and it is the subject of this book.

Here, again, we must be more specific if we want to be able to offer a meaningful answer. "Cancer" is a term that embraces many types and stages of disease, whose common feature is that cells, again of many different kinds, are proliferating to an excessive degree and settling in places where they disrupt the normal functions of the body. Certain cancers may be more susceptible than others to mental influence (for instance, those known to be affected by hormones, which are in turn influenced by the mind, such as some breast cancers), and it almost certainly makes a difference whether a cancer is a single, primary tumour or a widespread, late-stage disease. The qualities of the person with the cancer may also be decisive, as we will see later.

EARLY HISTORY OF THE IDEA THAT MIND CAN INFLUENCE CANCER GROWTH

How did the idea that the mind can affect cancer arise in the first place? Most of the scientific or systematic clinical work has been done only in the last 4 decades or so. This has never been a popular area of scientific study, in the way that, for example, immune responses to cancer or the impact of diet on cancer incidence have been, probably because it has been perceived as both difficult and somewhat radical.

Very few scientists have devoted any substantial part of their careers to it, funding has been hard to get, and progress therefore slow. Even within the area, most workers have confined their investigations to possible links between certain types of personality or mental state and the onset or progression of cancer, and only a minority have directly addressed the more practically important issue of using the mind as a potential therapeutic tool to affect cancer progression.

I am going to discuss first some earlier, exploratory studies, done between about 1960 and 1985, work that is now not considered definitive for technical reasons, as will be briefly explained. However, it has prompted a great deal of speculation in the popular press and media, which have seized upon the idea of a mind–cancer link, often simplifying and exaggerating it to a point where orthodox physicians and researchers have tended to dismiss the whole notion in angry reaction.

Modern views on the possible connection between mind and cancer can be traced back to Sigmund Freud, who proposed that unconscious mental conflicts could be expressed as symptoms in the body. A number of psychoanalytically oriented psychiatrists have since speculated that this kind of mechanism might be responsible for some cancers, which would provide a rationale for using psychotherapy as a treatment. Few professionals now give this idea much credence, however; the whole notion of bodily ailments as expressions of mental conflict is unpopular today (although the specialty field of psychosomatic medicine deals with some unarguable examples of mentally induced body symptoms, such as certain patterns of anesthesia, skin wheals, and others). If the mind-cancer-psychotherapy field has a "father," he would probably be Lawrence LeShan, a New York psychologist, who conducted scientific experiments in the 1950s suggesting that a severe loss or bereavement could prompt subsequent development of cancer. This idea has been reinvestigated a number of times since, without any consensus being reached. LeShan is a scholarly and wide-ranging thinker who in recent decades has not been much involved with the scientific community but has addressed himself directly to interested laypersons in a number of valuable books.

One of the latest is *Cancer as a Turning Point*,[2] whose main theme is that people with cancer may benefit most from pursuing not what is "wrong with" them (as tends to happen in conventional psychotherapy), but what particularly excites and interests them. Cancer is seen as an opportunity or motivating circumstance, time to reappraise life and make important changes. This idea occurs frequently, often in distorted form, in New Age publications.

The group that has perhaps had the greatest influence on the views of the general public toward mind and cancer was headed by Carl Simonton, a radiation oncologist, who worked with Stephanie Mathews-Simonton and James Creighton, and was associated with colleagues Jean Achterberg and Frank Lawlis. During daily relaxation periods, this group advised patients to imagine their immune defence systems overcoming the cancer cells in their bodies. The imagery chosen by patients was sometimes quasi-realistic, for example, white blood cells engulfing cancer cells, and sometimes more symbolic, for example, large dogs, representing the defences, eating up piles of meat (the cancer). Personal responsibility for healthy habits, the development of goals, and other lifestyle adjustments was also advocated. The book by the Simontons and J. Creighton *Getting Well Again*[3] has had a wide audience among people concerned with cancer. Drs. Achterberg and Lawlis also contributed scientific papers and books to the area, and Jean Achterberg has since written a number of more general books demonstrating the wide-ranging importance of mental imagery. The Simonton group found that the median survival time for patients taking part in a program using their approaches (in conjunction with conventional medical treatment) was about twice that of people with similar diseases at several major U.S. treatment centres. Critics have been quick to point out that one cannot infer, from this, that the imagery-related treatment caused prolongation of life, since the patients coming to the Simonton clinic were a highly selected sample—more motivated, better educated, and wealthier than average—and might have done better than most patients anyway. I would agree that this criticism is technically correct, although it does not *disprove* that the effect was real, and we will see in chapter 5 that the size of the effect they observed was similar to what we saw in a more controlled experiment.

Two rather similar accounts appeared at around the same time as the Simontons' (late 1970s and early 1980s). Bernauer Newton and his team[4] showed that of 105 cancer patients studied, those who received 10 or more sessions of psychological therapy that employed hypnosis were likely to live much longer than those who had fewer therapy sessions. Again, unfortunately, to draw definite conclusions from such an experiment it is necessary to demonstrate that the groups getting more or less help had disease of equal seriousness, and this was not done. In another study, Ainslie Meares,[5] an Australian psychiatrist, used intensive daily meditation with 73 cancer patients and reported complete remission of the disease in 5 of them, with 5 more having some remission of growth "in the absence of any organic treatment which could possibly account for it." He also published detailed case studies of some of his patients who survived unexpectedly. As for the Newton experiment, an unbiased reader would have to say that this is very interesting, but that independent data is needed to support the claim that this minority of patients would not have survived anyway.

These were all quite large studies, aimed at testing whether a psychological intervention could prolong the life of cancer patients. There were other accounts of similar attempts during this early period, but less systematic in character. At the same time publications were appearing on possible associations between patients' personalities and their survival; we will consider these in the fourth chapter.

CLAIMS IN POPULAR BOOKS AND THE MEDIA, AND THEIR IMPACT ON THE COMMUNITY

Over the last 2 to 3 decades a swelling flood of popular books has appeared offering medical and psychological advice to people with serious health problems, advice that ranges in value from helpful to questionable to downright dangerous (in the last category would be advocacy that a cancer patient should never accept chemotherapy). Some of the best of these works are by physicians or other health professionals who have become disenchanted with the exclusively materialistic emphasis of modern medicine and attempt to offer a more holistic approach (involving the patient's mind and spirit as well as the body). Many of them have been highly influential among people with cancer, although they are generally disliked by mainstream medical professionals. The main reason for this negative reaction is probably that the reality is much more complex and uncertain than it is made to appear.

Lay people reading books of this kind can gain the impression that by being optimistic, being in control, being active, making a decision to love themselves, they are likely to get well again. While there is some truth behind that view, as we will see in chapters 5 and 6, the claims are often sweeping and based on impressions, rather than evidence. Impressions can easily be mistaken; for example, when a scientific analysis of groups was conducted according to the principles espoused in *Love, Medicine and Miracles*, by Bernie Siegel,[6] participants failed to live longer than people in a comparison group who did not attend.[7] Errors commonly found in these more popular accounts include misconceptions about the state of research in mechanisms of cancer control; for example, attributing a major role to the immune system—a position that immunologists have not supported for at least 2 decades. There are often claims about powers of the mind that may be latent within us, but that almost none of us can exhibit, such as the ability to direct chemotherapy to a cancer or divert blood and starve a tumour. The psychological qualities of people who are likely to develop cancer tend to be spoken of as established, whereas scientists who have actually studied this issue are much less certain; see for example, the work discussed in chapter 4. Researchers who spend many years painstakingly dissecting complex questions like these have a right to be resentful about sweeping claims. In a related manner, the qualities that characterize survivors are often confidently asserted, on the basis of impressions, and on non-rigorous studies by others (which we will examine in chapter 3). The reality is again more complex. The implication that cancer patients often unconsciously "need" their illness is also a common claim that is unsupported by evidence, and is insulting to many. Books that uncritically extol the power of our mind may inspire hope, but they may also provoke despair. Two colleagues of mine, Brian Doan and Ross Gray,[8] have described the guilt and disillusionment that many of their patients feel when they try to live up to such recommendations, yet find that their cancer continues to progress.

It is, of course, particularly appealing to cancer patients to read accounts of patients who have unexpectedly recovered from serious disease, especially if that condition resembles their own. There are two main categories of books of this kind: studies by health professionals of patients who did well (chapter 3); and what we might call the "heroic survivor" accounts. The latter describe, usually in great detail, the struggles of an individual with his or her disease (cancer seems to attract more of these accounts than other diseases, in part because it is so often resistant to medical treatment). Such books can inspire hope and can reassure the reader that it is humanly possible to triumph, in spirit at least, over such severe challenges; the reader, whether lay or professional, can only respect the author's courage and resourcefulness. The danger in such accounts comes when it is stated or implied that what the writer did was what caused him or her to survive beyond medical expectation. We will meet this logical error again, in studies of remarkable survivors, but briefly, just because one person survived longer than predicted, and also engaged in some practice thought to be healing (perhaps followed a special diet), it cannot be inferred that the diet *caused* the long survival. We never hear from the many people who adopted the same diet and failed to survive! However, the stories may well point to healing strategies that deserve further investigation. I'll briefly mention now several books of this kind that, in my opinion, are responsible and helpful.

Claude Dosdall was a hospital administrator who developed a brain cancer, which was presumed fatal, but inspired him to investigate all aspects of his life and make changes. He lived for 10 years longer than predicted, and in that time founded an organization in Vancouver called HOPE, which offered support and education in self-help to thousands of people with cancer, and continues to operate long after his death. Claude's book, in typical humorous fashion, is entitled *My God, I Thought You'd Died*,[9] which is what a friend said on meeting him some time after his diagnosis!

The Five Stages of Getting Well, by Judy Edwards Allen,[10] is another example of the best kind of survivor book. At the age of 40 she contracted a breast cancer that spread and became incurable, and, like Claude, she examined all aspects of her life and changed them to aid healing. Judy described how she gained a great deal from a profound spiritual text *A Course in Miracles*, and she passes on to others the understanding that she came to on the surrender of personal, ego-driven ambition as a route to healing.

The book by Alice Hopper Epstein, *Mind, Fantasy and Healing*,[11] is unusual and fascinating. She recovered from a kidney cancer that had spread to the lung, in parallel with undertaking an inner journey to become acquainted with aspects of her personality that she "saw," in her imagination as little figures. There was "Baby Alice," a child representing the author's fearfulness; a crab that later turned into a bird, representing aspects of her relationship to a mother who would not "let her fly"; then "Amanda, the builder," a source of strength; "Little One," a volatile, feisty, personification of the author's hostility; and finally "Mickey," a complicated little girl who was a manifestation of jealousy. Alice (the author) had various imaginary encounters with these sub-personalities, which she came to understand and accept as outlets for emotions and behaviours that were difficult to express in real life. The figures all changed and matured during the course of her therapy with someone who must have been a very enlightened and supportive therapist. A single story does not constitute proof (in this case, that such imagery work can affect cancer progression), but an account like this does bring to our attention a possible route to healing for some people that obviously deserves much more investigation (there have been no such studies published, to my knowledge, since Alice's book appeared in 1989).

Finally, Ian Gawler, a veterinarian, wrote *You Can Conquer Cancer*[12] some years after surviving a malignant bone cancer that had spread to his lungs. Ian and his wife Gayle explored many unconventional routes to healing (conventional medicine had no cure for him), including attending meditation sessions with psychiatrist Ainslie Meares, whose study was mentioned earlier. His recovery seems truly remarkable: Dr. Meares published photos of Ian with bony growths in the lungs that protruded through the chest wall; Ian himself says he was spitting out bone at the time! However, he became healed, and has since devoted himself to running a large centre for cancer patients in Australia.

In addition to books such as these (and there are many more), one finds, sometimes it seems in almost every issue of certain popular magazines, accounts of people who "beat" cancer or another serious disease. These accounts are usually simplistic and often misleading. They may sell magazines, but they have the unfortunate effect of causing many health professionals to lump together and dismiss all attempts to study the potential of mind to influence healing of physical disease. Funding thus becomes difficult to obtain, and young investigators are discouraged from entering the field.

One very positive and concrete result of popular books and articles, however, is increased public awareness of the unmet needs that cancer patients and others have for emotional support. Community organizations may be set up to provide it; I've already mentioned the Gawler and HOPE centres. Often, as in these cases, it is the experience and drive of one dedicated survivor that stimulates the creation of such an institution; Gilda's Club, fuelled by the energy of a well-known comedienne, Gilda Radner, is another example. In my city of Toronto, Canada, the Wellspring organization was set in motion by Anne Gibson, who became enthusiastic after attending our Healing Journey program (chapter 5); Wellspring has since expanded to a number of other communities. Sometimes a centre will be initiated by people who have not themselves suffered from cancer but have become convinced of the value of such support; the Wellness community for cancer patients, founded by Harold Benjamin, has been a very successful example of this kind, with many centres now in the United States.

REACTIONS OF THE ORTHODOX
HEALTH CARE PROFESSIONS

In spite of the obvious value that cancer patients place on the support they get at community centres like these, this kind of care is not yet strongly advocated by many oncologist physicians. We can only speculate why this is so, in the absence of any in-depth investigation of physician attitudes. In part it may be a carryover of historical beliefs. Until 30 or 40 years ago in North America (and still in some European countries, apparently), physicians seldom informed their patients of a cancer diagnosis. This reticence was no doubt kindly meant—sparing the "victim" distress in her last months—but today it seems patronizing and misguided. At the very least, patients need the opportunity to plan their remaining time, if death is inevitable, and those who are interested in doing so should be given the chance to help themselves. More recently, around the 1970s, there was much argument about the value of support groups, where cancer patients could meet with one another and a leader, to share feelings and experiences. Those objecting claimed, presumably without the experience that would likely have convinced them otherwise, that such interactions would be depressing; for example, that if a group member died, it would harm other members emotionally. A small group of psychiatrists and psychologists showed that such was not the case, and argued for more open communication and emotional support for cancer patients generally; these included Irvin Yalom and David Spiegel of Stanford University, Jimmie Holland of the Sloan Kettering Institute, New York, William Worden and Avery Weisman of Project Omega at the Massachusetts General Hospital, and others.[13] This battle is now won: it seems incredible, in retrospect, that it could ever have been the subject of dispute. There is now ample empirical evidence to bolster the commonsense idea that emotional support is valuable for many cancer patients. However, by no means all express a wish for it, and why many don't is a question that needs in-depth investigation. Part of the reason is certainly unawareness of what group support can do, and apprehension about the benefits of talking frankly to other people with similar disease.

Although emotional support may be accepted, if seldom strongly advocated, by professionals, a further possibility is less widely accepted: that patients can do more than share experiences and emotions; they can learn active coping strategies, like thought management, deep relaxation, and meditation. Some of us who have explored these methods claim first that they can almost always help people cope better with the stress of cancer; and second, if they are pursued in depth (chapter 5), they may affect its course. While most oncologists, if pressed, would probably acknowledge the benefits of stress reduction, even this relatively conservative goal is not highly valued, judging by the scarcity of referrals and relevant programs. (Support groups are quite common in cancer centres, while programs teaching such active strategies are not). There is good evidence now that learning psychological skills helps patients enjoy a better quality of life, better in fact than simply meeting for support alone. Resistance may stem in part from lack of familiarity with the benefits of such help, coupled with a fear that it may lead patients to believe that the work can actually prolong their lives. And it is this second potential goal of self-help philosophy that, even when not openly expressed, raises fears among many professionals. Their frequent objection is that if anyone suggests that what we do with our minds might affect cancer (practising internally assisted healing, in our terminology), that suggestion generates "false hope," presumably meaning hope the speaker believes is unwarranted. For example, a committee examining the Simontons' work published a critique that simply dismissed their very interesting clinical observations, rather than seeing them as a basis for further investigation.[14]

SOME COMMENTS ON "FALSE HOPE"

Since the value of "hope" is presumably not really in dispute, a more accurate term would be "false expectations." It is undoubtedly true that irresponsible advice—whether for psychological techniques, diets, other unconventional remedies, or even conventional medical treatment itself—can stimulate unwarranted or unrealistic expectations. For this reason, and in pursuance of honest communication generally, doctors tend to be conservative (patients would often say "pessimistic") in their claims. There is a cost to such pessimism: I have heard over and over again from patients complaining that what their doctors told them "robbed them of hope" or "plunged them into despair," often by saying something like "There is nothing more we can do." There is always something that can be done for people, if "only" psychological and spiritual support, and communications can be put in a more positive way without being dishonest; for example, "There are no known cures for your kind of cancer at present, Mrs. X, and you must be prepared for the possibility that you will die, but there is always room for hope; new remedies are constantly being tested, and I've seen occasional individuals live for many years with what you have."

As a guide to presenting psychological approaches to helping oneself both feel better and perhaps live longer, I would offer the following suggestions. First, the professional can only advocate what he or she understands and believes, on the basis of thorough examination, to have some support from scientific evidence or systematic clinical observation. (Usually there is some degree of uncertainty, and this should be conveyed to the patient). It is dishonest to make claims that one can't support, but it is also dishonest and prejudiced to dismiss or disparage possibilities of which one has no experience, when there is some evidence for their value. Second, on the patient's side, the advice given should be only what that individual can understand; it has to make sense to her. Thus it is irresponsible to say to someone, "You must just love yourself and all will be well," if she doesn't have the remotest idea how to accomplish such a feat. Yet the same advice, coupled with psychotherapeutic help, might be valuable to a person who is able to see its point.

Current widespread medical resistance to the notion that patients can be taught to help themselves by psychological means may have deeper roots than "false hope." The view, which is an old one, that we can determine our biological destiny by voluntary means, to at least some extent, contradicts the whole philosophy of modern medicine, which is based on materialism. It regards the body as a machine, whose parts can be fixed from the outside by trained experts, and in which a mind exists somewhere but is largely isolated from the host body. However, buried within us all is a knowledge of potentials of this kind that we rarely access; health care professionals, like other people, have a distant intuitive awareness of these potentials, but are generally not trained to use it. Thus a sense of guilt, inadequacy as a healer, may often be present below conscious awareness, and may provoke an over-reaction when the possibility of mind–body healing comes up.

SUMMARY

Healing is broadly defined as restoration of, and ultimately improvement in, harmony, balance, and optimal functioning, within and between all parts of the person: body, mind, and spirit. It may be brought about by external agents and procedures ("externally assisted") or by changes from within a person's own mind ("internally assisted"). The latter is the main subject of this book.

We briefly explored early history of the idea that psychological healing methods could affect the progression of cancer, which has been widely advocated in the popular media but is still largely rejected by conventional medicine. Stimulating "false hope" is often cited by professionals as a damaging consequence of advocating use of the mind to assist healing; I suggest that such advocacy must be guided by knowledge of relevant evidence, without prejudice in either direction. What a professional can do for her patients in this way will depend upon both her understanding and that of the person receiving the assistance.

REFERENCES

1. Two books by the author designed to help cancer patients help themselves:
   Cunningham, A. J. (2000). *The healing journey: Overcoming the crisis of cancer.* (2nd ed.). Toronto: Key Porter.
   Cunningham, A. J. (2002). *Bringing spirituality into your healing journey.* Toronto: Key Porter.
2. LeShan, L. (1989). *Cancer as a turning point.* New York: Dutton.
3. Simonton, C., Matthews-Simonton, S., & Creighton, J. L. (1978). *Getting well again.* New York: Bantam.
4. Newton, B. W. (1982). The use of hypnosis in the treatment of cancer patients. *American Journal of Clinical Hypnosis, 25,* 104–113.
5. Meares, A. (1980). What can a patient expect from intensive meditation? *Australian Family Physician, 9,* 322–325.
6. Siegel, B. (1986). *Love, medicine and miracles.* New York: Harper and Row.
7. Morganstern, H., Gellert, G. A., Walter, S. D., Ostgeld, A. M., & Siegel, B. S. (1984). The impact of a psychosocial support program on survival with breast cancer: The importance of selection bias in program evaluation. *Journal of Chronic Disease, 37,* 273–282.
8. Doan, B. D., & Gray, R. E. (1992). The heroic cancer patient: A critical analysis of the relationship between illusion and mental health. *Canadian Journal of Behavioural Science, 24,* 253–266.
9. Dosdale, C. (1986). *My God I thought you'd died: One man's personal triumph over cancer.* Toronto: McClelland and Stewart–Bantam.
10. Edwards Allen, J. (1992). *Five stages of getting well.* Portland: Lifetime.
11. Hopper Epstein, A. (1986). *Mind, fantasy and healing: One woman's journey from conflict and illness to wholeness and health.* New York: Delacourt.
12. Gawler, I. (1984). *You can conquer cancer.* Melbourne: Hill of Content.
13. Holland, J. (1990). Historical context. In J. Holland and J. H. Rowland (Eds.), *Psycho-Oncology.* Oxford: Oxford University.
14. A critical editorial on the idea that mental techniques can affect survival:
    American Cancer Society (1982). Editorial. *CA: A Cancer Journal for Clinicians, 32,* 58–61.

Chapter 2

A Wider View: Can the Mind Heal the Body?

In this chapter I attempt to show that a case can be made for a mind–body link in many areas of health and disease. Against this background, it becomes reasonable to propose that cancer is in no way exceptional, and that the mind might affect cancer growth. The chapter is unavoidably more technical than the others in this book, although I've tried to make the discussion as simple as possible. I'll be introducing a way of thinking about the relationship between mind and body that is common sense and easily understood by anyone familiar with computers. However, readers who don't doubt the mind–body connection and who have little interest in the mechanisms by which it operates could bypass this chapter, or read only the first part of it; all subsequent chapters will be much more digestible for the layperson.

BRAIN AND MIND

The human brain is obviously a highly complex organ—in fact, it has been described as the most complex known structure in the universe.

This complexity grew as animals evolved; we can see anatomical evidence of, for example, the "reptilian brain" within our own. The function of the brain is to provide an overarching control of virtually everything that happens in the body. Lower levels of the brain, the "older" parts of the organ, maintain our blood pressure, heart rate, and breathing, and influence movements of our digestive system and much of the hormonal activity in our bodies. All of this would continue if we were in a coma.

With evolution came the ability to take some voluntary control over our actions, beyond reflexive responding. More elaborate functions depend on the cerebral cortex in the brain, and as this part developed, the ability emerged for communication through symbols, principally speech, and hence for reflective thought. Partly as a result of our more complex brains, and partly because of our cultural achievements, we humans have the capacity for sophisticated thinking including self-awareness and ability to manipulate and respond to abstract symbols and ideas ("mother," "love," "guilt").

The brain exercises its control over the body through physical pathways. A brain-initiated action begins when nerve cells, called neurones, "fire" (produce electrochemical impulses) in some part of the cortex. This activity spreads through various parts of the organ: the brain cells are all interconnected in a huge web or net. From the brain, nerve impulses may be passed down the spinal cord and along nerves issuing from the cord, to muscles or other organs in the body. A thought, in physical terms, is simply a particular pattern of nervous activity in the brain. How these physical events give rise to the experience we have of conscious awareness nobody really knows. Some nerve firings lead to sensations, like pain, others lead to thoughts.

This is where we come to the difficulty many medical scientists have with the idea that the mind might influence disease. Nobody has trouble believing that a *physical* event, like lots of nerves firing, has an impact on other parts of the body. But the mind, a *psychological* experience? How could such an intangible thing exert force on concrete structures in the body? In spite of the fact that we all know that a thought or intention can lead to immediate physical action, I think that the apparent incompatibility of thoughts and physical events has deterred many from taking seriously the possibility that mind could affect disease. The solution is clear: "thoughts" and "nerve cells firing" are just two ways of describing the same thing. They are two different languages, if you like (I discuss all of this more fully in a journal article cited at the end of this chapter).[1] "Mind," the sum of our thinking and sensing, is like software in a machine whose hardware is brain and body. We can influence the workings of a computer by making small physical adjustments to its internal wiring, but it is a lot easier and more efficient to operate through the software. Analogously, much of what the body does can be manipulated through the software of the mind. In the case of deciding to move a limb, we all know this. In the case of changing the course of a disease, we have barely begun to explore the potential.

Of course the body is a very complex machine, many of whose functions have evolved to function automatically without deliberate mental input, and will continue to operate in animals or people in a coma. Furthermore, some parts of the body are much more directly affected by the mind than others. As in the example just cited, we translate an idea into muscle action very easily and skilfully. Other parts are less accessible. Few if any of us can alter our heart rate simply by issuing an internal command to the heart. However, we can all learn to do it indirectly—by vividly imagining a frightening scene, for example. In recent years it has been found that many parts or functions of the body can be influenced that were previously thought to be entirely outside voluntary control. When I began research in immunology 40 years ago, the immune system was held to be quite autonomous; now we know it is very sensitive to psychological states, and that in fact the nervous and immune systems communicate constantly. On a more mundane level, distribution of blood flow seems to be quite readily affected by the conscious mind—this may be what Bernie Siegel was referring to when he suggested, as reported in chapter 1, that we have the potential to deliberately starve a tumour of blood. He may be right; it needs and deserves investigation. We do know that, with training, using techniques like biofeedback and hypnosis, most of us can learn some control of heart rate, blood pressure, skin temperature, patterns of electrical activity in the brain, even the firing of individual nerve cells. A beginning level of control over muscle tension allows people to achieve a depth of relaxation that they may never before have experienced (see chapter 5). And in people who have devoted time and study to personal control, remarkable feats have been documented, like enduring large puncture wounds from metal skewers without subsequent bleeding or infection.[2] No doubt there are many barriers to direct translation of thoughts into physical change in the body, but there are ways around some of these barriers.

To summarize, in terms of theoretical possibilities, once we recognize that "mind" and "brain activity" are two ways of describing the same thing, it is no longer surprising that we might have the potential to affect many body functions through conscious thought. And in terms of practical evidence, we already know that sophisticated mind–body connections can be made, even if they are not within the repertoire of most of us as yet. It seems important to keep an open mind, and to explore further.

PATHWAYS CONNECTING MIND AND BODY

Just as we can decide, in examining the brain, to focus our analysis either on its detailed anatomical mechanisms or on the way information is passed through it, so we can look at mind–body connections in terms of mechanisms of information transfer. The former is what usually has been the concern of medical scientists. The latter, focusing on the "logic" of the connections, will be more useful to us here, and has the advantage of being readily understood without a technical background.

A diagram will show how the mind transmits "messages" that promote or heal disease (Figure 2.1). Events in our environment, meaning social interactions and life circumstances generally, are perceived and appraised by us in ways that depend on a host of factors, such as our cultural background, our individual history, the context

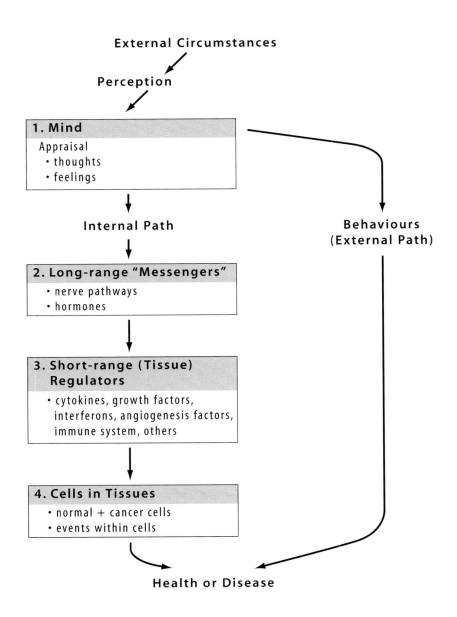

FIGURE 2.1 *Some of the steps in the "internal" path between events in the mind (thoughts, feelings, perceptions) and their ultimate impact on bodily health.*

of the events, and our state of mind at the time. Perhaps the most basic appraisal is, "Does it threaten me, or does it seem desirable?" This appraisal, in combination with other mental events of which we are unconscious, determines our emotional reaction (experienced as a "feeling" in both mind and body). This is the most crucial step in the chain (and, incidentally, the one over which we can exert most voluntary control). I've shown it as a "mind" box. Thoughts can be viewed as packets of information.

As a result of these events in the mind, messages are sent to all parts of the body. It is important to distinguish two kinds of result, as in Figure 2.1: externally observable behaviours that indirectly affect health, and internal changes that do so more directly. These correspond to the externally and internally assisted healing routes of chapter 1. Nobody doubts the external route of disease causation. For example, a frequent appraisal such as, "I can't stand this situation, pass me the bottle," might lead to developing a harmful addiction. The external/behavioural path to causing disease might involve smoking, overeating, alcoholism, failure to exercise, non-compliance with medical advice, dangerous driving, and many other kinds of behaviour. If the appraisal is, "I have a disease, I need to do something about it," then the external loop on the diagram represents externally assisted efforts to heal the condition, such as seeking medical advice, taking medication, adopting healthier habits, and so on.

The "internal" path refers to changes in distant parts of the body as a direct effect of messages generated in the mind/brain, not mediated through externally observable behaviours. This is what is usually meant by "healing through the mind," and provides another route through which the onset or progress of ill health might be deliberately affected. In broad outline, as we react psychologically to our environment through our thoughts, we signal the body to be prepared to adapt accordingly. For example, a perceived threat might stimulate a raised heart rate, tensing of muscles, and other expressions of readiness for action. This signalling is done through two major channels: the nervous (electrochemical) system and the endocrine (hormonal, chemical) system. The electrical or chemical signals are physical in nature, but carry information, just as an electrical signal in a telephone wire may do. This long-distance communication (acting over the whole extent of the body) affects specific tissues; in our example, a signal to prepare for action, transmitted down a chain of nerve cells, could cause muscle fibres to contract. The long-range signalling systems, though nerves and hormones, affect the local systems of regulation in most organs of the body.

These processes of local regulation, which I've labelled "short-range messengers" in the figure, have the task of maintaining healthy functioning in their immediate vicinity. It is an axiom of modern biology that virtually all cells in the body are constantly being acted upon by their neighbours and by molecules (hormones, nutrients, other signals) in the fluids that bathe them. Cells that divide frequently, like those in the lining of the gut or parts of the skin, are in particular need of constant monitoring and control of this kind, or they will simply continue to divide, and may generate cancerous tumours. We will discuss later in the chapter the little that is known about the mechanisms by which incipient cancerous growths are controlled. To anticipate the later discussion: we now know that cancers emerge not only because the cells comprising them are genetically abnormal, but also because of some failure of this local regulation.

As the final step in the pathway, I've shown a box for the cells that are the target of all this control or regulation: this includes both normal (dividing) cells and cancer cells. To sum up this section then, messages originating in the brain/mind affect, through long-range and short-range messenger-regulators, the behaviour of cells in most tissues of the body; if this regulation is impaired, disease may follow.

DIFFERENT DISCIPLINES STUDY DIFFERENT "BOXES"

The diagram also helps us see why the division of mind from body has been perpetuated, and, I hope, how we can begin to heal the breach. Biomedical science as I've said is concerned mostly with mechanisms, particularly at the bottom of the pathway. This focus has led to an understanding of the cellular and molecular changes accompanying disease, and has often allowed development of procedures and drugs to reverse some of these changes. For example, if we observe that plaque builds up in coronary arteries and may block them, provoking heart attacks, this leads to surgical methods of treatment; when the biochemical basis of plaque development is understood (for example, the contribution of excess cholesterol), drugs are designed to counteract the problem.

When we look at box 1, however, we enter a territory in which the appropriate research methods, and even the language, are quite different; it is the province of health psychology and mind–body medicine. Psychologists have to observe what is going on in the mind/ brain indirectly, relying on subjects' self-report and behaviours, then describe this in terms of "information," that is, as patterns of words and actions, rather than in structural or biochemical terms (while modern neurology is developing scanning methods to detect activity in the brain, they detect only relatively gross changes). These patterns can then sometimes be related to ultimate health or disease. The social determinants of health-related behaviours are also of interest to health psychologists, and draw upon a further set of concepts; to know how to induce young people not to smoke, for example, we need to understand not only individual psychology but also the culture that encourages this behaviour. The situation is similar when helping people change such behaviours as abusing alcohol and drugs, overeating, practising unsafe sex, driving danerously, even committing suicide.

In this book we are mainly concerned to examine aspects of box 1 and test their impact on progress of disease. Don't we need to know all the intermediary steps, as some researchers insist, before we accept that mind and body are, in fact, connected? This is not logically necessary: if we find a consistent pattern of thought and behaviour associated with a disease, and if changing the mental state corrects the disease, we have the required evidence. Furthermore, the events connecting mind/brain and body are so complex that complete understanding is still a long way off. Most researchers are fully extended learning the concepts and methods in one part of a single box, and have to rely on other specialists for information about the rest. Of course it is always valuable to know as much as possible about the pathways by which a treatment works; our knowledge is obviously more complete if we can say, "The psychotherapy produced a drop in levels of circulating stress hormones, and enhancement of immune function, and as an apparent result, a clearing of the infection"! We will have a brief look at what we know of such mechanisms later in the chapter. One value of a detailed understanding is that we can begin to use drugs to repair the ravages of unhealthy thoughts and behaviours or to substitute for healthy mental change (a mixed blessing, however; for example, over-reliance on analgesics like Aspirin may prevent us from recognizing behaviours that are ultimately self-destructive; furthermore, most drugs have unwelcome side effects).

MIND AFFECTING HEALTH AND DISEASE: EXAMPLES

We will look briefly now at the evidence for involvement of mind in a number of specific symptoms and diseases. This is not intended to be a technical or definitive review. My purpose here is to provide an overview showing that the contribution of mind is already known in many cases. It will also become clear that illnesses can be placed on a spectrum: those with obvious psychological links at one end, and those where any mental involvement is relatively obscure at the other. I've clustered diseases or symptoms into three broad categories, based on the degree to which this link is manifest.

The evidence for involvement of mind, where it exists, is of two main kinds: observations showing that a condition is prompted or made worse by state of mind (usually "stress" in some form), and evidence that psychological intervention alleviates the problem. The first kind is much more common, I think, because the usual conservative view of health scientists is that we need to see evidence for a connection before being justified in trying mental remedies. In fact, alleviation through psychological change is the most practically useful, and often the most powerful, evidence one can get for a mind–disease link.

Conditions Where the Mind–Body Link Is Obvious, and Alleviation or Reversal Is Clearly Possible through Mind

Many of the conditions in this cluster are not dramatic, yet together they are probably responsible for the bulk of the health-related suffering in the world (at least in those countries where famine, war, or endemic plagues are uncommon).

We can start with the suffering brought about by what I will call "harmful self-talk." Anxiety, sadness, anger, and much depression are to a large extent a result of such self-talk, although it is common to blame external circumstances, such as difficulties in relationships, for our unpleasant thoughts and moods. They can bring about such "physical" symptoms as fatigue, headaches, insomnia, sexual dysfunction, and disturbed appetite (I use quotation marks to highlight the artificiality of the distinction between "physical" or "organic" on the one hand and "mental/psychological" on the other). Many of these problems can be alleviated by a shift in patterns of thinking—assisted, where necessary, by psychotherapy—which can help us see that it is not our circumstances but mental reactions to them that cause distress. The Buddha pointed out this fact 2500 years ago! Much the same applies to unhealthy addictive behaviours such as smoking, using street drugs, drinking alcohol, practising unsafe sex, overeating, even driving unsafely or risking trauma in dangerous occupations and sports. This is not to claim that shifts in perspective are easy—often they are not, and harmful habits of thought and reaction may become ingrained as a result of early life experiences and later reinforcement. Nevertheless, the possibility of reversing them by mental means exposes their psychological origins. Clinical depression, one of the most widespread and costly disorders in the modern West, is sometimes represented as an "organic" problem (several types are recognized by experts), implying that it was visited upon the sufferer, with no contribution from his mind or behaviour. It is true that there is a biochemical basis for the disease (as there is for all functions of mind)—for example, there may be insufficient amounts or inadequate distribution of certain neurotransmitters (chemicals) in the brain. However, this defect may often be restored either by drugs or by psychotherapy,[3] the latter route producing the longer-lasting effects, as the depressed person learns to control his own mood. For some other serious mental diseases—schizophrenia, for example—it does appear that there is no realistic possibility of voluntary control, and that drug treatments are the only choice.

Chronic pain, often without obvious physical causes, is another example of a condition that seems to be "physical" in origin, yet it can be both exacerbated and alleviated through the mind. It afflicts millions of people—chronic low back pain, for example, is the leading cause of workplace disability in the province of Ontario, Canada. Both medical and lay people tend to act as if such pain were susceptible only to physical remedies, but there is abundant research to show that psychological methods can often alleviate it.[4] For example, a panel of experts brought together by the American National Institutes of Health, whose findings were published in the conservative *Journal of the American Medical Association* in 1996, concluded that "a number of well-defined behavioral and relaxation interventions now exist and are effective in the treatment of chronic pain and insomnia."[5] It also noted that this approach to therapy is seldom employed.

"Stress" is a useful term for a definite state of reaction in body and mind to challenging circumstances (usually it occurs when we are afraid we can't cope with a situation). The external circumstances are the "stressors," our *reaction* the stress. Being or feeling stressed seems to make us more vulnerable to many medical conditions. For example, susceptibility to the common cold has long been associated, in folklore, with stress. So it is gratifying to see evidence for it, in an article published in a prestigious medical journal in 1991 by Cohen, Tyrell, and Smith.[6] Just under 400 subjects were inoculated with cold viruses, and it was found that the likelihood of contracting an acute respiratory illness increased in proportion to the degree of stress subjects were experiencing in their lives (assessed using a series of question-naires). Some other common infectious illnesses (that is, caused by micro-organisms) are also acknowledged to occur more often or with more severity under stress, such as those caused by the herpes viruses (cold sores, genital herpes, shingles), some fungal infections, some types of viral hepatitis, and HIV-AIDS.

It is probable that stress promotes infections, by diminishing our immune responses to the foreign organisms.[7] Other important conditions that are not caused by viruses or bacteria are also widely acknowledged by experts to be worsened by stress, such as hypertension (elevated blood pressure), which is a risk factor for heart attacks. On the "healing" side, there is evidence that psychological treatments such as relaxation training decrease the risk of heart attack. There is also abundant evidence that psychological interventions can speed healing after surgery.

Social circumstances, acting through the mind (through our perception of their importance to us, and the emotions they invoke, the top box in Figure 2.1), are a potent source of both stress and healing. There is a consensus on the life-sparing benefits of good social support, and on the harmful effects of social isolation (as may occur following bereavement, for example). More dramatically, it has been well documented that people whose life expectancy is short tend to live until important anniversary dates, such as their birthdays or other culturally significant dates, and then die soon afterwards.[8] And on the other side of the coin, equally dramatic, is the phenomenon of "voodoo" or "hex" death, where anthropologists have described the deaths, within days, of members of a tribe who were placed under a lethal curse or spell by their witch doctor.

In summary, we already know that many of our most prevalent health-related problems in the West are largely induced by our minds (that is, by patterns of thinking), and can be alleviated or cured by changes in the mind. This being so, it would seem logical, as many writers in this field have noted, to use therapy or treatment at this level (Figure 2.1, box 1) to solve the problems.

Conditions Where There Appears To Be a Contribution by Mind, although Less Widely Acknowledged

This category overlaps with the last, and includes many important diseases for which there is some evidence that the mind plays a role (internally promoted or assisted). Medical opinions vary (the evidence is seldom irrefutable); more materialistically oriented physicians focus entirely on physical aspects of cause, while health psychologists and more holistically oriented physicians see a contribution from the mind. In almost all cases, however, standard treatments are physical (external) in nature.

A list of the major conditions would include: myocardial infarction (heart attacks), peptic ulcer (but see below), and chronic disorders of the bowel like irritable bowel syndrome and Crohn's disease, bronchial asthma, rheumatic diseases and arthritis, some dermatological conditions like psoriasis, endocrine disorders like diabetes mellitus and thyroid disease, infectious diseases, including those mentioned in category 1 above, progression of AIDS, autoimmune diseases, such as lupus erythematosus, and others.[9]

Let us look at some examples from this list. Coronary heart disease (blockage of coronary arteries leading to heart attack) is the leading cause of death in Western cultures. While diet and exercise play a role, there is a large body of research demonstrating that hostile thoughts and feelings translate into higher susceptibility to this disease (and probably to many other serious illnesses). The evidence is strongest for the consistent *association* of hostility and anger with incidence of heart disease, but there are also intervention studies, showing that incidence of disease and death can be substantially reduced by teaching people how to reduce time urgency, competitiveness, and hostility, and replace them with beliefs and behaviours rooted in patience, tranquillity, and empathy.[10] A determined critic can say, however, that the counselling did not produce an "internally assisted" healing, but acted solely by changing the behaviours of the individuals whose health improved, for example, by persuading them to adopt healthier habits (externally assisted healing).

It is probable that both paths of pathogenesis (disease production) and healing are involved in many diseases, as is well illustrated when we consider another important chronic condition, diabetes mellitus. To slow the progression of this disease and avoid serious complications, like blindness or loss of limbs, it is vital to have good management of blood glucose levels, which requires a disciplined regime of insulin injection, and also control of diet and exercise. Maintaining adequate self-care behaviours is usually dependent in turn on a healthy emotional state and good support from family and medical teams. In other words, the internal state influences the external/behavioural loop. In addition, there is undoubtedly a direct, internally mediated effect of mind, through emotional state, on blood glucose levels and carbohydrate metabolism generally. Emotional stress mobilizes blood sugar, and periods of relaxation and rest can decrease the amount of insulin needed. Similar remarks would apply to many chronic diseases: there is a need for behavioural management, and also a likely direct effect of mental-emotional state on the disease. Peptic ulcer, for example, has long been attributed to stress; the recent discovery of a bacterium as a causal agent does not disprove the importance of mental state, but rather shows that several factors are important, including mind. In a similar way, any widespread outbreak of infectious disease always fails to affect a proportion of the population, and mental factors are likely to be among the reasons for this resistance.

An example of mind acting in a beneficial way through internal mechanisms only, comes from the healing of wounds. There is consistent evidence, in both animals and humans, that stress of various kinds slows wound healing significantly. Conversely, healing after surgery is accelerated by psychological stress management. A second example is the intriguing recent series of experiments showing that simply writing about stressful life experiences relieved anxiety, and provided prolonged relief of symptoms from two "physical" conditions: rheumatoid arthritis and bronchial asthma.[11] A third example is the phenomenon of classical conditioning, familiar to all through Pavlov's dogs, who learned to salivate at the sound of a bell, which had become associated with the expectation of receiving food. We humans do this too—try imagining a delicious apple pie, baking in the oven! We are conditioned in many ways to respond bodily to things our minds perceive. Classical conditioning—for example, automatic fearful responses to some stressors—undoubtedly plays a role in health and disease. In all these cases the pathway from mind to body appears to be purely internal.

This brief discussion will have given some indication about the difficulty of establishing a direct influence of mind on disease. Modern medical theory is very materialistically oriented, preferring to find objective, external causes for illness. Faced with evidence for a role of mind, a materialist's next line of defence is to insist that the mind is not really acting internally, but merely instructing the body's musculature to act in certain ways, to bring helpful external agents to bear. The interested reader might like to consult a fascinating exchange, published in *Psychosomatic Medicine*.[12] Two protagonists, Redford Williams and Neil Schneiderman, argued that there was good evidence for mind–disease links, and gave examples. Two others, Arnold Relman and Marcia Angell, both eminent members of the American medical establishment and editors of the prestigious *New England Journal of Medicine*, disputed this evidence. Several things emerge from this debate. First, its polarized, antagonistic tone (a far cry from disinterested seeking for truth). Second, the *New England Journal* people have a point: irrefutable evidence is hard to come by. Third, there is a deep ideological resistance, masquerading as scientific rigour, to seriously considering a significant role for mind in disease, at least in some quarters. Dr. Relman is quoted as saying, "The power of mind and thought to change physical matter and heal organic disease [is] a concept which basically contradicts the laws of physics in the modern scientific view of nature." In other words, he has overlooked the fact that information affects matter, which we see all around us, in the workings of our computers as well as in our bodies.

Does it matter whether mind affects disease through external or internal routes or loops? Perhaps not to the suffering individual who, in a given instance, simply wants relief. But the distinction is important for its impact on our research and treatment methods. To the extent that we deny mind, we will focus on ever more elaborate external, technical methods for treating disease. At the same time, we take away from the individual what is possibly a considerable potential to help herself. We will come back to this crucial point at a number of places later in this book.

Conditions Still Usually Thought To Be Independent of Mind

Most experts in cancer medicine or research would place the disease in this category. All acknowledge that the majority of cancers are mentally induced through the "external" pathway, by unhealthy behaviours, notably smoking and poor diet. However, the internal pathway, the person's thoughts and feelings, are not generally considered to have any potential direct effect, either in causing or alleviating the disease (we will examine this further in subsequent chapters). In fact, cancer research seems to be focusing more and more on the genetic changes that cause cells to become potentially cancerous. While most cancers seem to arise as a result of spontaneous changes in the genetic material of a single cell after birth, in other cases people inherit specific defective genes that make development of cancer very much more likely. It is now estimated that 5% of all cases of newly diagnosed breast, ovarian, endometrial, colorectal, and prostate cancers are inherited in this way. For example, in the case of breast cancer, two such genes (BRCA1 and BRCA2) have been identified.[13] Somewhat more than half of the women inheriting defects in one of these genes will get cancer (unless the breasts are removed as a preventive measure). Of interest to us here, however, is that not all women who have these genes do get cancer—other factors, possibly including the psychological, must also be operating. This highlights a more general principle. Although cancer is often described as a "genetic disease," and diseases caused by micro-organisms as "infectious diseases," all maladies are the result of contributions from all of the "levels" we portrayed in Figure 1.1. There are always social influences (for example, choice of a mate in genetic disorders, local sanitary conditions in an infectious disease), always physical factors, and inevitably always psychological influences acting either through behaviours, or by what I've called the internal route, or both.

What about the fact that animals get many of the same kinds of disease we do (as a former veterinarian, I am particularly aware of this)? Does it not disprove that mind is necessary? And what about diseases in very young children; how can their minds have had time to contribute? I would respond that mind can have an impact only to the extent that it is developed in an individual, animal or human. I am not arguing against the importance of genetic or other physical/biological determinants of disease, but am simply saying that when a conscious mind exists, it will inevitably exert a effect on the more automatic functions of the brain, and hence on the body (see next section). This will both foster disease and provide an avenue for alleviating it in many cases. However, when a person is born with a disease, genetically induced or otherwise, direct effects of her own conscious mind can presumably be ruled out. An example is Huntingdon's disease, caused by a single gene, whose inheritance invariably brings about brain degeneration and death, the symptoms usually beginning in mid-life, although even here, the variable age of onset points to an influence of factors other than the purely genetic.

SOME MECHANISMS BY WHICH MIND IS
KNOWN TO INFLUENCE DISEASE

We have couched our discussion to this point in terms of the flow of information from one part to another, rather than in concrete terms of molecules, and nerves firing. As pointed out earlier, the *logic* of the interactions is more important to our purposes here than the detailed mechanisms. Once we know that certain kinds of message undermine or promote health, we can immediately apply this knowledge, like operating a computer from a knowledge of the logic of its software, without needing to know the electrical and mechanical basis for its operation. However, it is reassuring to know something about the molecular and cellular events that carry these messages. Let us therefore have a brief look at the nature of the long-range messages influencing health, about which quite a lot is known, then at controlling cancer growth through short-range messages, which are still poorly understood.

The Mind and Long-range Messengers

The mechanical connections between the body and the aware or conscious mind are of three kinds. The first is called the voluntary part of the nervous system. Ideas or sensations in the mind, which are a reflection of masses of nerve cells (neurons) firing in the cerebral cortex, can be directly channelled into messages (electrical impulses, generated in turn by flow of certain molecules called neurotransmitters) down specialized motor neurons in the spinal cord and along the nerves leading to our "voluntary" or striated muscles, meaning most of the large muscle groups. We decide to move, we move, thanks to this chemical flow of intention. Second, and distinct from all of this, is the involuntary or autonomic nervous system, which controls the functions of organs other than the striated muscles. Thus autonomic control (involving both "sympathetic" and "parasympathetic" parts, which balance each other), affects heart rate, patterns of blood flow, respiration, digestion, liberation of energy molecules from the liver, aspects of sexual behaviour, and other functions. This more primitive part of the nervous system also interacts with the endocrine or hormonal system, which constitutes a third major link between mind and body.

When we are "stressed"—whenever there is a challenge of any sort, any perception of events requiring a response beyond the most routine—our minds must decide how to react. The most basic kinds of reaction are what the famous medical researcher Walter Cannon called, in the early 1900s, "fight" or "flight." As we realize that a response is needed, two main sets of events take place: first the sympathetic nervous system sends nerve impulses to the heart, increasing the rate of its cycle of contraction, and to blood vessels, directing blood to the muscles, and to the energy system, mobilizing glucose. It also sends impulses to the core of the adrenal glands, situated above the kidneys on either side of the body. These glands then immediately secrete adrenaline, which increases the general arousal. Simultaneously the endocrine system contributes directly: as the perception of threat or challenge filters through various levels of the brain, it reaches the hypothalamus, which is a primitive part controlling most hormonal activity. The hypothalamus signals the pituitary gland, sometimes called the master gland, which is situated beneath it. This gland, in turn, releases hormones into the blood that can have many effects, particularly on other glands in parts of the body like thyroid, pancreas, and testes or ovaries. During the response to stress, the most important hormones from the pituitary are those that stimulate another part of the external part of the adrenals, to release corticosteroid hormones. These also have widespread effects, for example, on inflammation and on the immune system (see below).

This is a bare outline of the stress response, but if it seems technical, the important point is that we know how thoughts and feelings in our conscious minds can induce profound changes in the rest of the body through these long-range messenger nerves and molecules. It thus makes biological sense to speak of mind affecting the body. We also know that if this sort of adaptive response is provoked continuously over a long time, harmful effects on many of the body's organs are likely. The exact pattern of such breakdown varies from person to person, depending on their physical status, their coping resources, and other factors.

Short-range or Local Messengers, and Local Control of Cancer

The control of the growth and differentiation of dividing cells of many kinds, including cancer cells, is an exceedingly complex process. Research on it is currently fragmented into many specialized area, and integrative reviews are difficult to find. What follows is a tentative outline. In general, we can say that the local environment in which a cell finds itself is very important in determining whether and how often it can divide, whether there is a change in character of the progeny as they divide and multiply, and whether or when the cells finally die. The immediate neighbours of a given cell exert an influence. Locally produced protein molecules called growth factors or cytokines bind to its outer surface, the resulting balance of positive and negative signals determining whether or not division occurs.

The development of clinical cancer usually begins with a mutation, a change in the genetic material or DNA, of a single cell. When this cell divides, some of its progeny may undergo further changes, giving rise, after months or even years, to a family of cancerous cells that are less susceptible than normal cells to local control mechanisms—hence their dangerous tendency to proliferate in an unrestrained way. Many types of dividing cells in the body, such as skin, muscle, various glands, lymphocytes, bone, blood-forming cells, and supportive tissues in the brain (but not the normally inert nerve cells), may undergo this kind of transformation, leading to the more than 100 kinds of cancer that are currently described. Cancer cells also may produce molecules that promote the development of blood vessels around the growing tumour, which is limited, as are normal tissues, by the supply of available nutrients. As these pathways become better understood, this knowledge should suggest biochemical ways to control cancer. Exploration of possible therapeutic effects of some of these regulator molecules has already begun: lymphokines, a type of cytokine produced by lymphocytes, have shown promise in treating malignant skin cancer and renal cancer, and another class of regulator molecules called interferons, which are made by a variety of cell types, has also proved to have anti-cancer activity.

Another type of regulator that has long been investigated for its powers to control both infectious disease and cancer is the immune system. It is really an organ in itself, but one whose cells are not in constant contact with one another; many of its cells, the most important being lymphocytes, circulate freely around the body, while others, such as macrophages and dendritic cells, are often stationary, and line vessels within lymph nodes, the spleen, and other organs. Among the lymphoctyes are a category called cytotoxic (cell-killing) T lymphocytes, which are able, under some conditions, to attach to and destroy cancer cells. This potential is also exhibited by other cells of the immune system at times, including so-called natural killer cells, although their clinical importance is not yet clear. Lymphocytes also produce lymphokines, as just discussed, and these molecules can enhance the cytotoxic effects of other lymphocytes. One effect of mind on the immune system that is quite well understood is that if a sense of threat or stress is persistent, it causes lymphocytes to be shunted out of the blood circulation, and hence to be less available to fight infectious disease or cancer. While the immune system undoubtedly is a major mechanism for controlling infectious disease, its importance in cancer control is much more doubtful: for example, if it were crucial, we would expect that experimental animals born without a functioning immune system would quickly succumb to one of the common cancers, but this is not observed. This is a pity from the point of view of those of us wishing to argue that mind may affect cancer, because it is now well established that mind events, such as the perception of stress, may significantly depress immune responses! In the mind–immune system–cancer pathway, then, the second link may not be of much clinical significance.

What evidence is there that mind-stimulated changes in the long-range messengers influence patterns of local control of cell proliferation in a way that might affect cancer? To my knowledge, there is very little such evidence yet in terms of detailed mechanisms. However, we can make quite a strong case on more general grounds. First, the passage of information or messages from a central organizing system (brain, nervous system, and endocrines) to local environments, is simply the way the body works. (It is also the way any organized entity, such as a complex machine, or a corporation, works.) More specifically, certain common observations on the behaviour of cancers imply that they, like all other dividing cells, are not autonomous but are subject to at least some regulation, and where there is regulation there is potential mental influence. For example, when autopsies are done on people dying of non-cancer causes, a high incidence of small, precursor cancers is found in tissues like breast or prostate, many more than would ever have become clinical tumours. These must have been controlled in some way while the person was alive. A related observation is that some cancers, notably those originating in the breast, may remain dormant for a long time, even decades, then suddenly appear at multiple sites. Something must have held them in check during that time. Spontaneous remissions are occasionally seen (see next chapter), implying regulation, without indicating how it may have occurred. Many cancers are sensitive to natural hormones such as estrogen, allowing for mental influence, since all such hormones are affected directly or indirectly by the mind. There is other, more technical evidence, which in sum is sufficient to convince cancer scientists and clinicians that the old view of a cancer as an autonomous invader, immune to local conditions, is incorrect. However, while most would now agree that the development of clinical cancer is caused both by genetic changes in the cancer cells themselves, and with a failure of the host to regulate the growth of those cells, few would yet consider that the mind of the host matters very much, once cancer has been found, which is, of course, the case I am trying to make in this book.

HEALING THROUGH SYMBOLS

These last two sections will be more speculative. I will outline a way of interrelating and understanding several puzzling phenomena, such as the role of expectancy in healing, the power of suggestion, and possible effects of spirituality on healing.

Let us start with the placebo effect, which is a phenomenon very familiar to Western medicine.[14] Placebos are substances or procedures without known specific activities, which nevertheless cause healing change. The actual agents may be sugar pills, injections of distilled water, sham surgeries, physical manipulations, prescribed diets or other regimens, even conversation with someone assumed to have answers for the sufferer. The common factor seems to be that the agent has *meaning* for the patient; it or he or she is a *symbol*, something that stands for something else, in this case, for a potential transition to a healed state. Placebos affect many kinds of physical condition, such as pain, breathing problems, fevers, skin conditions, and wound healing. They can also induce negative physiological states, like weakness, nausea, rashes, or pain. These effects are not "all in the mind"; actual physical change can often be seen and measured, as, for example, when such interventions have been shown to stimulate production by the brain of endorphins, substances that help the body control pain. The proportion of those treated showing effects from a placebo varies, in different studies, from 10% to 90% (and is commonly around 30%). Modern trials of new drugs almost always include a placebo control, meaning patients who receive, without knowing it, an inert substance in place of the active drug; specific activity attributable to the drug is then considered to be any effects it produces over and above what the placebo does. At times the placebo is as effective, or almost as effective, as the drug! This phenomenon is clearly an example of the mind affecting the health of the body.

The placebo effect is the best-studied of a group of phenomena that may in fact all have a similar basis. In brief: an object, person, or procedure acts a symbol, inspiring hope, and perhaps mobilizing normally dormant potentials, in a person desiring healing. Thus the symbol *suggests* to the sufferer that healing is possible, and the suggestion brings about mental changes, which in turn stimulate beneficial physical change.

We can list a number of examples where suggestion, or placebo effect, appear to be operating. Symptoms can be induced by suggestion; at a mundane level, most of us are familiar with feeling nauseated by thoughts of revolting foods or activities. The psychiatric literature describes patients who display symptoms for no known physical reasons, symptoms like strange patterns of pain or anesthesia, paralysis, false pregnancies, and others. Conventional research methods have established that positive expectancy is associated with better outcomes in cancer, HIV-AIDS, and other diseases. Faith healing, which seems to promise miraculous cures by charismatic figures, is probably a form of suggestion. In earlier and less technological societies, the healer was often a shaman who would manipulate objects and perform procedures that seem quite irrational to modern Western people, yet at times alleviated disease. The wide variety of special diets and injectable substances offered to cancer patients and others by non-traditional therapists seem to be an example of remedies related to those used by shamans, and likewise capable of inspiring hope, if not physical cures (research is needed to test whether such agents do have a placebo effect in cancer). Hypnosis can be characterized as a procedure that helps patients suspend their normal, rational way of experiencing the world, leaving room, as it were, for new potentials to be activated. Even social support may act in part through suggestion, by creating in the sufferer a sense of being cared for, of being important to others. Dramatic examples of the impact of suggestion, already discussed, are voodoo death (a negative placebo), and the way people are sometimes able to postpone their death until an important date has been reached. And finally, self-image, which is in turn largely created through interactions with others, also has a potent impact on both the care that a person will take of herself and on the whole range of thoughts and emotions she has about her prospects for recovery and her life generally.

All of these phenomena appear to be mediated by symbols to which the person in distress attaches significance and emotion. These symbols are manipulated or changed during the healing ceremony or interactions: the witch doctor shakes his animal skulls, the community rallies around and expresses caring, the faith healer performs a ritual, the modern physician brings high-tech apparatus and powerful drugs to bear, the unconventional dietitian proposes a diet that, it is claimed, "has cured others." The patient ideally becomes an active participant in, and subscriber to, the process of manipulating the symbols, and invests time, belief, and often money, in them. She then sees the operation of the symbols as an indicator of actual change in herself. To put it another way, change in the symbolic world has spoken deeply to the mind of the patient, and allowed her to change her perception of the real world. To the extent that mind does affect body, this symbolic process may actually cause change in health status.

This process is well known to anthropologists (see, for example, an article by J. Dow).[15] It would probably appear fanciful to many

Western-trained health care professionals. However, the power of suggestion is susceptible to scientific investigation; placebo research is a good example of such work. Note that it does not require any esoteric mechanisms, anything thought intrinsically impossible by the laws of physics—simply a relaxing of the severe limitations that the biomedical world currently places on the effects it deems the mind can have on the body. As we turn now to the final section we will, however, touch on realms beyond the strict Newtonian universe that still informs most theory-building in health care.

SPIRITUALITY AND HEALING

Religious and spiritual ideas and experiences have been important to many suffering people throughout human history. I will return to this point in a slightly different way in chapter 7, but for the present we need to define the two labels: "religion" refers to an organized social structure of belief and ritual; "spirituality" refers to an individual's experience of being connected in some way to an order, intelligence, or divine being that transcends the material world, and is all-embracing. The two terms, formerly closely related, are now increasingly differentiated, although both describe aspects of the human search for ultimate purpose or meaning.

To portray the various ways in which either religious observance or spiritual experience might affect health, I have added another box to our earlier diagram (see Figure 2.2). A sense of connection to a transcendent order might influence behaviours, such as self-care, that contribute to externally assisted healing. Alternatively, it could exert an influence through the internal pathway, by enhancing a person's sense of hope, or of being loved and worthwhile. In this way it might resemble social support in its effects. A third possibility is more radical: spiritual connection might have a direct impact on the body and on health, by mechanisms unknown.

Research on the relationship between spirituality and healing is at an early stage, just coming out of the closet, so to speak. To take the spiritual dimension seriously it is probably necessary to have one's

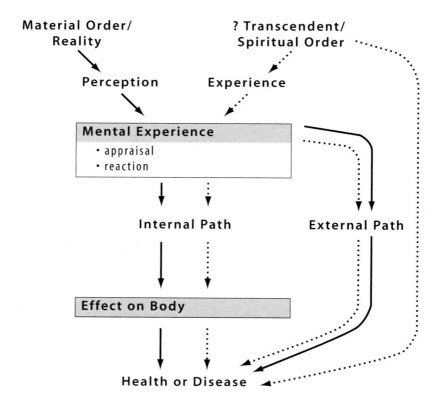

FIGURE 2.2 *Three ways in which spiritual phenomena or experiences might affect health: by changing thoughts and feelings in a way that leads to either behavioural change ("external path") or an alteration of "internal pathways"; or alternatively, by some direct—as yet unknown— mechanism, independent of thought.*

own experience of it: without this experience, the ideas can seem absurd; with it, there is no doubting its central relevance and meaning in life. However, objective scientific study of a possible relationship to health can be carried out by treating spirituality in the same way as any other set of psychosocial variables, which usually means giving subjects one of the available questionnaires, and relating their responses to some measure of health status. There are a lot of studies showing that religious observances, such as attending church or synagogue, correlate with enjoying better than average health, but authors are always careful to point out that this could be a result of healthier behaviours—our "externally assisted" pathway—or simply a reflection of the fact that people who are intrinsically more healthy are more likely to attend church. Little has been done to assess the impact of deep, personal, spiritual experience on health. Particularly needed are systematic longitudinal studies (that is, following people over time as they receive training or therapy and develop their spiritual awareness). There are already many anecdotes relating improvements in health to development of a spiritual connection, as we will see in the next chapter. There has also been some research on 12-step programs for addiction, which certainly help at least some participants, and have a strong spiritual component.

Surprisingly, some recent, technically sound studies support the existence of a direct influence of prayer on health, through what appears to be an example of the third pathway shown in Figure 2.2: a direct link between the spiritual dimension and the body. Two large, randomized controlled trials (see chapter 4 for an explanation of this technique), have demonstrated that there is a significant tendency to recover better from a heart attack when the patient is prayed for, without his knowledge, by other individuals who did not know him and had only his name and a few other details to "direct" their prayers. There are some other smaller positive studies of the same kind, and also some that gave negative results. Analyses of the field as a whole conclude that there is likely to be a real effect; it is easy to imagine ways in which such studies could fail to produce a result, but very difficult to see how a "false positive" could occur. This is indeed a puzzling phenomenon, inexplicable by current theories.

SUMMARY

It can help us understand the often contentious idea that an intangible "mind" affects a concrete "body" if we consider a computer analogy: mind is like the software of a computer, and body the hardware. Mind–body connections can thus be described either in terms of the passage of information, or as physical mechanisms. A mental appraisal, such as response to threat, sets in train two kinds of event: first, an external pathway of behavioural change, and second, an internal path comprising a definite series of "messages" to many parts of the body, the messages being carried by quite well-understood nervous and hormonal pathways.

We surveyed the evidence that mind can promote disease, noting there is a spectrum of conditions ranging from those obviously mind-influenced, like clinical depression, to others, like coronary heart disease, where the connection is highly probable, if not universally accepted, and to still others, like inherited genetic disorders, where there is presumably no such effect. We looked also at some of the related but scantier evidence for the power of mental change to alleviate disease.

Finally, we considered evidence for the effect of symbols, such as placebo treatments, acting through the mind, to influence the body, and for the possible routes by which spiritual experience or connection might affect health.

REFERENCES

1. A discussion of how thoughts can be viewed as the software that influences the physical hardware of the body:
   Cunningham, A. J. (1995). Pies, levels and languages: Why the contribution of the mind to health and disease has been underestimated. *Advances: Journal of Mind–Body Health, 7,* 41–56.

2. A review of the research studying effects of meditation in expert meditators:
   Davidson, R. J., & Harrington, A. (Eds.). (2001). *Visions of compassion: Western scientists and Tibetan Buddhists examine human nature.* Oxford: Oxford University Press.

3. A review of the efficacy of psychotherapy in the treatment of depression compared to anti-depressant medication:
   Antonuccio, D. O., Danton, W. G., & DeNelsky, G. Y. (1995). Psychotherapy versus medication for depression: Challenging the conventional wisdom with data. *Professional Psychology: Research and Practice, 26*(6), 574–585.

4. Johnson, W. G., Baldwin, M. L., & Butler, R. J. (1998). Back pain and the need for a new paradigm. *Industrial Relations, 37*(1), 9–34.

5. NIH Technology Assessment Panel on Integration of Behavioral and Relaxation Approaches into the Treatment of Chronic Pain and Insomnia. *Journal of the American Medical Association, 276,* 313–318.

6. Cohen, S., Tyrrell, D. A., and Smith, A. P. (1991). Psychological stress and susceptibility to the common cold. *New England Journal of Medicine, 26,* 309–322.

7. Kiecolt-Glaser, J. K., McGuire, L., Robles, T. F. & Glaser, R. (2002). Psychoneuroimmunology and psychosomatic medicine: Back to the future. *Psychosomatic Medicine, 64*(1), 15–28.
   Marsland, A. L., Bachen, E. A., Cohen, S., Rabin, B., & Manuck, S. B. (2002). Stress, immune reactivity and susceptibility to infectious disease. *Physiology and Behavior, 77,* 711–716.
   Stowell, J. R., McGuire, L., Robles, T., Glaser, R., & Kiecolt-Glaser, J. K. (2003). Psychoneuroimmunology. In A. M. Nezu, C. M. Nezu, & P.A. Geller (Eds.), *Handbook of psychology: Vol. 9. Health psychology.* New York: John Wiley & Sons.

8. Phillips, D. P., & Feldman, F. A. (1973). A dip in deaths before ceremonial occasions: Some new relationships between social integration and mortality. *American Sociological Review, 38,* 678–696.

9. Any comprehensive textbook on health psychology will review the relevant research linking psychological factors and various diseases and conditions. Two such texts are:
   Bellack, A. S., & Hersen, M. (1998). *Comprehensive clinical psychology: Vol. 8.*

Health psychology. D. W. Johnston & M. Johnston (Vol. eds.) Oxford: Elsevier. Nezu, A. M., Nezu, C. M., & Geller, P. A. (2003). *Handbook of psychology: Vol. 9. Health psychology.* New York: John Wiley & Sons.

10. Krantz, D. S., & Lundgren, N. R. (1998). Cardiovascular disorders. In Bellack, A. S. and Hersen, M. (Eds.). *Comprehensive Clinical Psychology: Vol. 8. Health Psychology.* D. W. Johnston and M. Johnston (Vol. eds.) Oxford: Elsevier Press. Rozanski, A., Blumenthal, J. A., & Kaplan, J. (1999). Impact of psychological factors on the pathogenesis of cardiovascular disease and implications for therapy. *Circulation, 99*(16), 2192–2217.
    Ornish, D. M., Brown, S. E., Schwartz, L. W., et al. (1990). Can lifestyle changes reverse coronary disease? The lifestyle heart trial. *Lancet, 336,* 129–133.

11. Smythe, J. M., Stone, A. A., Hurewitz, A., & Kaell, A. (1999). Effects of writing about stressful experiences on symptom reduction in patients with asthma or rheumatoid arthritis: A randomized trial. *Journal of the American Medical Association, 281*(14), 1304–1309.

12. Markowitz, J. H. (2002). Resolved: Psychological interventions can improve clinical outcomes in organic disease; Moderator introduction. *Psychosomatic Medicine, 64,* 549–551.

13. Lagarde, A. (2003). Genetics of common hereditary cancers. *Oncology Exchange, 2*(3), 8–37. Wooster, R., & Weber, B. L. (2003). Breast and ovarian cancer. *Genomic Medicine, 348,* 2339–2347.

14. A series of articles in *Advances in Mind–Body Medicine, 17,* 291–318. Also well discussed in Benson, H. (1996). *Timeless healing: The power and biology of hope.* New York: Scribner.

15. Dow, J. (1986). Universal aspects of symbolic healing: A theoretical synthesis. *American Anthropologist, 88,* 56–69.

Chapter 3

Studies on "Remarkable Survivors" from Cancer

Cancer is traditionally considered to be a group of diseases that progress inexorably and overwhelm the host unless the responsible cells are entirely removed. Yet some cancers, like lymphomas (cancers of lymphoid tissue) may pursue an erratic course, waxing and waning for years. Others—breast cancer is an example—may lie dormant for years, then suddenly appear and grow at many sites simultaneously. Occasionally, cancers regress completely without treatment, and this may be either temporary or long-lasting (many years, or permanently). This phenomenon has been called "spontaneous remission/regression," an unfortunate term, since it implies lack of cause, when in fact the cause is simply unknown. While dismissed by some, because it is rare and unpredictable, it has been hailed by others as an indication that some kind of internal control of cancer must exist, an understanding of which might lead to ways of boosting the body's intrinsic powers of resistance. It has been noted that certain types of cancer are more likely than others to disappear "spontaneously," for example, tumours originating in the kidney (hypernephroma) or skin (malignant melanoma). Possible explanations of the phenomenon have been framed almost entirely in terms of biological mechanisms: for example, activation of suppressor genes, hormonal changes, immune responses, or interference with nutrition (blood supply) of tumours. Some such process is presumably responsible at the tissue level, but the possibility that it is precipitated by an initial psychological event has rarely been considered.

People from whom all signs of cancer have disappeared in a lasting way, not attributable to medical treatment, or who have greatly outlived their predicted lifespan, are sometimes called "remarkable survivors"; they are the subject of this section. As in the last chapter, we are not as much concerned with the specific biological mechanisms that might bring about such remission as with the psychological patterns they display. If common features can be found, this suggests (although it does not prove) that adopting some of these attitudes might be protective in other cancer patients. It will also be interesting to compare the results of these studies with those obtained in the more rigorous experiments described in chapters 5 and 6.

HOW RELIABLE ARE STUDIES ON REMARKABLE SURVIVORS?

It would seem a commonsense notion that we could find what psychological qualities, if any, promote survival in patients with cancers that are normally fatal, by seeking out and interviewing individuals who survive much longer than expected. If we could identify some whose cancer had gone into complete remission, so much the better. However, there is one unavoidable and serious limitation to conclusions that can be drawn from this approach, which is perhaps why it has been seldom adopted by investigators. With a backward-looking design like this, we might find a particular pattern, say a strong fighting spirit, among remarkable survivors, but if we interview only these people, we cannot know how common this pattern was among those who failed to survive. To make this point more concrete, imagine that someone followed a diet consisting of nothing but grapes, and recovered from serious cancer. That individual is likely to swear that the diet cured him. Yet there may have been 100 or 1000 others who used the same diet but failed to outlive their prognosis. Against this background, the first individual would seem much less like a "remarkable survivor" and more like someone who was lucky for unknown reasons: perhaps his disease was misdiagnosed, or was less serious than was initially thought. Of course the diet (or the mental attitude, if that was the proposed mechanism of cure) *might* have been effective for him, but we can't be sure of that. For this reason, "prospective" studies are much more highly valued, meaning those in which we make the assessments of mental attitude, or diet, or whatever else we are interested in as investigators, *before* the survival outcome is known. This is likely to be difficult to do because, if an event is very rare, we may need to follow hundreds or even thousands of people in order to end up with one or two who show the phenomenon of interest, in this case lengthy survival (we will see in chapter 5 how this problem can be circumvented).

There are other technical problems with the available studies on remarkable survivors. In most cases, little effort was made to establish that the individuals did, in fact, have a medically incurable cancer in the first place; at times it is clear that some of them did not. And the methods used to describe their psychological attitudes usually have not come up to the kinds of standard required in modern medical-social research; the studies I will allude to are often more impressionistic than scientific. However, there is a feature of the studies in this field that may prompt even a skeptical reader to take them seriously: a remarkable consistency in the qualities reported among people who survived when apparently they should have died. We will look at the details of one of the studies, then put together a pattern emerging from them all. This analysis will later be compared with the results of the more rigorous prospective study described in chapter 5.

BERLAND'S 1995 STUDY

Berland's is one of the best of the small number of published studies; the author interviewed 33 individuals who had lived well past their medical prognosis, and reports his results as an indication of why these people believed they had survived, rather than as proof of qualities that promote survival.[1] In fact, this is all one can confidently deduce from data of this type; yet just beneath the surface, and of much greater interest, is the implication that these psychological qualities actually help people live longer. My critical comments here are intended to illustrate how difficult it is to draw this latter conclusion, by referring to limitations in this investigation and other similar ones.

Selecting subjects is the first requirement: 33 were obtained, more than usual in this type of study, mainly from physicians' referrals. Most had lived 5 years or more since diagnosis. Evidence of "remarkable survivor" status was simply an opinion from their health care provider that the chances of such lengthy survival had been considered small (less than 20% in all cases, less than 5% in 13 of them). No information was given on the types or stages of cancer. Without this reassurance, and without knowing the expertise of the health care diagnosticians (and even non-specialist physicians are unlikely to have a sound idea of probable survival times), we cannot have great confidence that each subject was suitable for the study. It is even possible that some had medically curable diseases, as was the case in some other reports of this kind. However, let us assume that most were relevant.

The next and most important task is obtaining from participants an account of what they believed was important to their recovery. All were interviewed and were also asked to list the activities and attitudes to which they attributed their recovery. This list of attributions provided some interesting results, in particular that spiritual, attitudinal, and behavioural qualities, plus support of family and friends, were viewed, on average, as twice as important as medical treatment! Only 5 of the 33 gave 50% or more of the credit for their recovery to medical or alternative material treatments. The interviews provided more data: unfortunately, little information is given about them beyond the statement that they were "structured and unstructured" (it is not clear whether each participant was interviewed once or twice). Tables are provided showing how many interviewees responded to questions about their attitudes and behaviours, although no detail is available on how what the subjects said was recorded and analyzed. The value of the study would have been enhanced by the use of well-developed methods of qualitative analysis, in order to draw inferences in as unbiased a fashion as possible from such interviews, as was done in some of the other similar reports. However, by an informal process Berland defined three categories of "survivor": 5 men with "fighting spirit," 10 participants who were "attitudinally and behaviourally focussed," and 18 who were "spiritually and existentially oriented." All but 5 of the 28 in the last 2 groups were women, an interesting fact in accord with our own experience that women are much more likely than men to try to help themselves psychologically against cancer (although there are exceptions, women tend to be more aware than men of what is happening in their minds and bodies, and less concerned with maintaining a facade of being in control).

The 5 men in the first subgroup differed markedly from the rest. They denied that the disease would kill them and professed a "fighting spirit." The other 2 subgroups exhibited quite a different range of qualities, and seem, to my reading, to have been quite similar to one another. Survival was attributed to taking an active role in changing attitudes and behaviours. There was a strong emphasis on learning to have one's own needs met, on an altered sense of self, and often on an increased connection with a spiritual source (especially in the third subgroup), all leading to a much improved, more secure, and emotionally authentic life (I offer below a more detailed "map" of the development of these qualities, taking all the studies into account). A characteristic statement by one woman: "It's the commitment, 100 per cent to never not live your truth . . . to live fully." The difference between subgroup 1 (the 5 men) and the rest is so marked as to suggest that, if survival was related to psychology for those in groups 2 and 3, this was not the case for the men in subgroup 1.

Berland provides an entirely reasonable and insightful discussion based on his findings. He points to the importance of attending to the psychosocial and spiritual issues that patients value, and describes similar findings made by others. Because of the technical limitations of this report, any implication that such factors are relevant to recovery is not likely to be taken seriously by researchers in the field of psycho-oncology or health psychology generally. This possibility does become more important when we relate Berland's work to that of other investigators, as we shall see.

AN INTEGRATION OF THE STUDIES ON "REMARKABLE SURVIVORS"

In preparation for writing this chapter I read or reread (having first done so 10 to 20 years ago) most of the available papers and books on this subject that seemed to have at least some pretension to objectivity. I had always tended to downplay the importance of this evidence, because of the technical problems we have discussed, particularly the issue of not knowing how many individuals displayed qualities like determination or recovery of self-esteem, but failed to survive. Yet on this rereading, I was struck by two things: first, by the agreement between accounts, and second—and to be honest, probably more strongly by—the concordance between these reports and what my team and I have found in the more rigorous prospective work in which we have been engaged for the last 10 years (chapters 5 and 6). I'll now try to draw the remarkable survivor studies together, and offer a scheme showing the relationship of the various qualities to one another, which has not, as far as I know, been done in this way before. The most important papers reviewed are by Ikemi, Nakagawa, Nakagawa, and Sugita, 1975[2]; plus some later unpublished work from this group; Achterberg, Mathews-Simonton, and Simonton, 1977[3]; Roud, 1986 (he has also published a book on his work)[4]; Huebscher, 1992[5]; Berland, 1995 (discussed above); and Denz-Penhey, 1996.[6] Two other reports of high quality available in unpublished form were from a group in the Netherlands by Schilder, de Vries, Goodkin, &

Antoni.[7] Of non-technical books, the most relevant is LeShan's *Cancer as a Turning Point* (see chapter 1). I also reviewed *Healing Yourself* by Pennington,[8] and (in part) *Remarkable Recovery* by Hirshberg and Barasch,[9] and a compendium of cases and commentary on spontaneous remission by O'Reagan and Hirschberg.[10] In a different category (much more definitive) is *The Type C Connection* by Temoshok and Dreher,[11] which will be referred to in chapters 4 and 6. Many more journalistic stories or anecdotes on this subject exist in the trade press; such casual, after-the-fact accounts are completely unreliable.

Figure 3.1 is an attempt to interrelate the principal psychological qualities described as associated with prolonged survival from life-threatening cancers. It is a dynamic model, in that certain attributes are proposed as leading to others, in other words as a hypothesis about the kinds of change that make survival more likely. There are 3 main parts. Starting qualities are those that a person needs to be able to initiate the deep psychological change indicated in the square box. These changes lead to the development of a second tier of qualities, 2 related, personal attributes, almost always described as prominent in people who outlive their life expectancy from cancer: autonomy, meaning the perception of having free choice of one's actions, and acceptance of self as worthy, as OK. The triangle formed by openness, leading through psychological change to increased autonomy and self-acceptance, lies at the heart of self-healing, at least as retrospectively described. The development of what we may call this "authenticity" of the self brings further benefits, shown under mental/emotional outcome at the bottom of the diagram: better relationships with others, often a shift towards a more spiritual orientation, and a zestful, more joyous appreciation of life. As these qualities develop, they encourage still more change; to keep the diagram simple, I haven't shown such positive feedback.

The starting qualities are hardly surprising. One needs openness or flexibility of views to contemplate change, coupled with a determination to do what one can to help oneself. This must in turn be supported by a belief, both in one's ability to make appropriate changes and in the methods employed. This pattern is in agreement

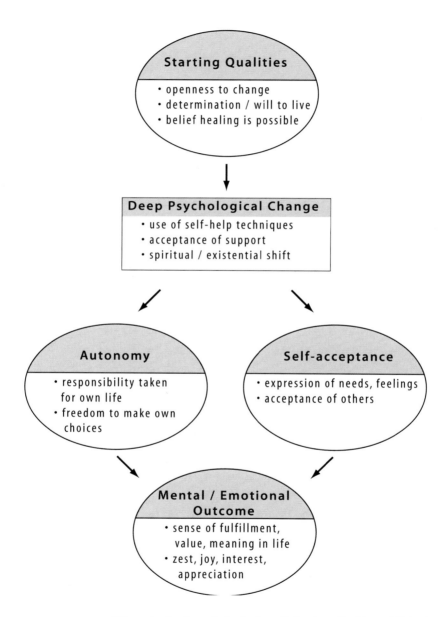

FIGURE 3.1 *The principal psychological qualities described in published accounts of "remarkable survivors," and the likely interrelationships between them.*

with a great deal of research on the process of change in other areas of psychology, such as the giving up of unhealthy habits. The specific methods that cancer patients used varied widely, often within a single report. Among the most common were meditation, prayer, affirmations, mental imaging, psychotherapy for insight, body therapies, and a range of alternative remedies ("externally assisted healing" in the terminology of chapter 1) such as diets and dietary supplements. The variety suggests that the specifics may be less important than the sense of control developed by using them.

The outstanding new qualities that long survivors reported in almost all studies were autonomy coupled with a better acceptance of self. They described becoming content with themselves: "I am who I am," as one participant related. This acceptance allowed, or was promoted by (the two categories in the diagram reinforce one another) the taking of more responsibility for one's life and living as desired, doing what one had always wanted to but had perhaps felt inhibited from pursuing because of a distorted sense of obligation to others. Now these obligations mattered much less; it was not so much a shedding of necessary roles as a healthy freedom to act upon what was felt to be best for oneself. As is well known in general clinical psychology, acceptance of oneself allows tolerance of the vagaries of others, and may lead to greater love and appreciation for them. Conflicts tend to be resolved in such a mental climate. Finally, for many but not all participants in these studies, there was what authors have often described as an existential shift, meaning a change in perception of one's relationship to the world, with greater sense of purpose or meaning in life, and often an increased spiritual sense of being part of a larger, non-material or transcendent order or God. Epiphanies, mystical experiences, or sudden transformations were not uncommon.

The overarching impression is that these people set themselves to combat their poor prognosis in a determined, energetic, and courageous way, and the result was what we might call a recovery or discovery of a more authentic self. Not surprisingly, life became much improved for virtually all of these people. A typical quote would be, "I'm just having the best time of my life!"

WHAT CAN WE CONCLUDE
FROM THESE STUDIES?

A skeptical person might say that the publications on remarkable survivors prove nothing, that the results can be explained in ways other than by assuming that the changed mental state caused regression of the cancer. Technically speaking, such critics are correct. It is possible that some other, unknown factor caused, simultaneously, the consistent change in psychology and the cancer regression. This was the kind of argument advanced for many years against the idea that smoking cigarettes causes lung cancer. Another objection is that these unusual people may have survived for purely biological reasons (perhaps the cancer was misdiagnosed), and the fact of surviving, being such a profound relief, induced the psychological change. This flies in the face of clinical experience: when people are let off the hook by a remission or cure of disease, the tendency is to return to old habits, to put it all behind them, and rarely to make the effort to maintain a changed life. We see this in many people recovering from primary cancers: the motivation for change is quickly lost. We would have expected a majority of remarkable survivors to show such unchanged patterns if the remissions were independent of mental state. Thus the most likely explanation is that profound psychological change, in the direction shown by these studies, promotes remission of cancer at times. One thing that these experiments cannot tell us, however, is the *frequency* with which becoming "authentic" promotes healing. It cannot be ruled out, from retrospective studies like these, that many more individuals made the same kinds of psychological shift but did not survive. A reasonable interim hypothesis would be that the mental changes make survival more probable, but that much depends on the nature of the specific cancer as well.

SUMMARY

Cancers very occasionally regress in the absence of any apparent physical cause. People who had a terminal diagnosis but whose cancers have gone into long-term remission have been interviewed in a number of studies aimed at relating psychological qualities and changes to the unanticipated survival. While such backward-looking studies are technically weak—since it is impossible to know how many individuals with similar psychological attributes did not survive—they have yielded highly consistent patterns. "Remarkable survivors" had common qualities that would assist change: openness or flexibility, determination to live, and belief in the possibility of their recovery. They reported substantial psychological shifts leading to a greatly increased sense of autonomy and self-acceptance—the freedom to live their lives as desired, rather than as constrained by imposed obligations. The changes also greatly improved the quality of emotional life, with joy, interest, peace, fulfillment, and zest for life being commonly reported.

REFERENCES

1. Berland, W. (1995). Can the self affect the course of cancer? *Advances: The Journal of Mind–Body Health, 11*(4), 5–19.
2. Ikemi Y., Nakagawa, S., Nakagawa, J., & Sugita, M. (1975). Psychosomatic consideration on cancer patients who have made a narrow escape from death. *Dynamic Psychiatry, 31,* 77–92.
3. Achterberg, J., Matthews-Simonton, S., & Simonton, O. C. (1977). Psychology of the exceptional cancer patient: A description of patients who outlive predicted life expectancies. *Psychotherapy: Theory, Research and Practice, 14*(4), 416–422.
4. Roud, P. C. (1986). Psychosocial variables associated with the exceptional survival of patients with advanced malignant disease. *International Journal of Psychiatry in Medicine, 16*(2), 113–122.
   Roud, P. C. (1990). *Making miracles: An exploration into the dynamics of self-healing.* New York: Warner.
5. Huebscher, R. (1992). Spontaneous remission: An example of health promotion. *Nurse Practitioner Forum, 3*(4), 228–235.
6. Denz-Penhey, H. (1996). *Poor prognosis, quality outcomes.* Unpublished doctoral dissertation, University of Otago, New Zealand.
7. Schilder, J. N., deVries, M. J., Goodkin, K., & Antoni, M. (2004). Psychological changes preceding spontaneous remission of cancer. *Clinical Case Studies, 3*(4): 288–312.
8. Pennington, S. (1988). *Healing yourself: Understanding how your mind can heal your body.* Toronto: McGraw-Hill Ryerson.
9. Hirschberg, C., & Barasch, M. I. (1995). *Remarkable recovery: What extraordinary healings tell us about getting well and staying well.* New York: Riverhead.
10. O'Regan, B., & Hirshberg, C. (1993). *Spontaneous remission: An annotated bibliography.* Sausalito, CA: Institute of Noetic Sciences.
11. Temoshok, L., & Dreher, H. (1992). *The Type C connection: The behavioral links to cancer and your health.* New York: Random House.

Chapter 4

Cancer and Mind: Current Scientific Views

In chapter 1 we took a snapshot of lay and professional attitudes to the idea that one's state of mind might affect the progression of cancer. The reader will have gathered that the lay enthusiasm expressed in certain quarters has not been matched by professional endorsement! However, having declared that there is a case to be made for a mind–cancer link, I embarked on an attempt to present this argument, beginning, in chapter 2, with some background evidence and ideas on the impact of mind on health generally. We saw that the mind is important in many disease processes, although there is as yet little effort to incorporate into the regular medical management of disease any mobilization of whatever potential patients may have to help themselves. Then in chapter 3 we examined the first kind of evidence relating specifically to cancer: interviews with remarkable survivors. The technical weakness of this evidence is compensated for to some extent by the very consistent picture that emerges from most of these studies: survivors demonstrate a pattern that I called "authenticity." In the present chapter we will examine the broader field of psycho-oncology, which is concerned with all aspects of the mind–cancer relationship, and see if research under this umbrella can shed any light on whether or not mental state influences survival from cancer.

PSYCHO-ONCOLOGY

This specialty area may be thought of as a branch of health psychology, or of "behavioural medicine" (whose main concern is, as the name implies, with the impact of behaviours on health). Psychooncology has recently been elevated into a vigorous and popular discipline in its own right through the efforts of a number of prominent clinical scientists, in particular Jimmie Holland, a psychiatrist at the Sloane-Kettering Institute in New York. A wide range of professionals work in the area including psychiatrists, psychologists, social workers, nurses, pastoral counsellors, and others.

Psycho-oncology is interested in both directions of the mind–cancer interaction: how having cancer affects mental state, and how events in the mind might affect cancer development and progression. The former has received much more attention, perhaps because it is easier to study; the extent and kinds of distress caused by cancer have been extensively documented. The ways in which oncologists and patients communicate is another important practical area that has been the subject of many papers. Much attention has also been given to developing self-report questionnaires to assess cancer-related distress—in part with the aim of efficiently detecting those most needing help. As one might expect, there has also been considerable work on how to alleviate this distress, an area that overlaps with our concerns here, and thus deserves some further discussion.

PSYCHOLOGICAL SUPPORT TO ALLEVIATE
THE EMOTIONAL STRESS OF CANCER

Cancer patients with severe depression, suicidal thoughts, or psychotic reactions, or who for other reasons find the diagnosis particularly difficult to cope with are often referred to mental health professionals for individual consultations, and possible psychiatric treatments (anti-depressant drugs, for example). However, the great majority of people who contract cancer are psychologically "normal," and able to handle the distress, although likely to experience additional anxiety and depression as a result of the diagnosis. In recent years, it has become quite common for community organizations and treatment centres to offer group meetings to support these people and their families through the crisis of cancer (similar groups also exist for people with other diseases). These support groups tend to operate outside the medical mainstream; that is, patients elect to attend them, and they are seldom a prescribed part of medical management of the disease. There is now good evidence that, as might be expected, attending such support groups helps relieve emotional distress and improve quality of life, although for many years this fact was not generally accepted by health care professionals, the concern being that contact with other ill people would be too discouraging or depressing for participants.

Participating in a support group—sharing experiences with others who are able to understand and empathize—is, in effect, a very basic way of enlisting potentials of the mind. It brings about some healing, in the sense of relieving suffering. Yet only a minority of people with cancer avail themselves of such support. Reasons for this reticence are unclear; it is a least partly due to lack of awareness of how sharing can ease distress, or fear of what a group discussion might involve. These groups can move beyond emotional support: a number of clinical scientists (including my own team) believe that they may, indeed should, incorporate training in active coping skills, as will be described in chapter 5. There is evidence that this helps patients more than support alone; for example, learning coping methods like relaxation has been shown to alleviate such symptoms as anxiety and depression, or the nausea that chemotherapy often induces.

RESEARCH IN PSYCHO-ONCOLOGY ON THE IMPACT OF MIND ON THE DISEASE

Although the main emphasis of psycho-oncology has been documenting and alleviating the mental distress that cancer causes, the possible impact of mind on the physical disease has also been considered. There have been two main kinds of investigation. The first really belongs to the broader field of public health, and is the study of behaviours that promote cancer, and how these behaviours may be modified. This is an example of what we described, in chapter 1, as the "external" route to causing or healing disease. In the modern Western world, most ill-health is now attributable to harmful behaviours, and in the case of cancer, it is estimated by experts that the incidence of disease could be reduced by about two-thirds through not smoking, making dietary change (avoiding obesity, high-fat diets, and excessive alcohol consumption), taking better care to prevent sunburn, avoiding environmental and industrial carcinogens (cancer-producing agents) like asbestos, and not engaging in unprotected sex with multiple partners (which can spread viruses responsible for AIDS and some gynecological cancers).[1] Perhaps the most important single contribution that could be made to cancer care would be finding a way to dissuade young people from taking up smoking. Not surprisingly, much research is devoted to this aim.

The second kind of research on mind affecting cancer is concerned with a possible "internal" route through which mind could influence onset of the disease, or affect its progression once acquired. This approach is not usually of interest to public health officials, but has a minority following, so to speak, in the subspecialty of psycho-oncology. There are what we may call descriptive and therapeutic approaches to this subject. The descriptive approach involves looking for relationships between mental qualities (often described as "personality") and the incidence or progression of cancer. Do people with certain psychological qualities tend to get the disease more often, and does the disease progress more readily in those with particular traits? We will look further at this question below, and I will try to explain why this kind of research has taught us very little. The therapeutic approach is the more obvious one: why not provide a psychological therapy to cancer patients, and see if they do better than a comparable group not receiving such help? This strategy has been explored much less than a lay reader might expect, given the obvious central importance of the question to psycho-oncology. We have already encountered some of the reasons for this modest exploration—basically, a cultural assumption that it's not possible, coupled with the (related) objection that one should not inspire "false hope" by making the attempt (chapter 1). However, in the last 15 years or so, there have been a number of experiments of this kind, which we will also examine in a moment.

RELATIONSHIP OF "PERSONALITY" TO CANCER ONSET AND PROGRESSION

The possibility of a relationship between aspects of one's personality and the risk of getting cancer has been a matter of fascinated speculation for at least a century, although reliable investigations extend back only for the last 30 years or so. A number of investigators (myself included) have published technical reviews of this literature,[2] but we need only a brief overview here. In a word, the results of this work have been disappointing. There is much inconsistency: research group A finds that stress of some kind promotes cancer, and group B then publishes a paper saying the opposite. This variability is presumably the result of different conditions between experiments: in the cancer patients involved, in their diseases, and in the measurement tools used. It is impossible to replicate studies with human beings exactly. No overwhelmingly strong associations have emerged between mental attributes (often loosely called "personality") and risk of getting cancer, or doing poorly once you have it. However, two factors do occur in a relatively consistent way in different studies. Repression of emotion, as a style of coping with problems in life, seems to favour cancer onset and progression (repression means that unpleasant emotions are blocked from awareness, and is more profound than suppression, where the person is aware of his or her deliberate non-expression). Secondly, having strong social support seems to be somewhat protective, as it is for many diseases. These results do *not* mean that, for example, an emotionally repressed person will necessarily contract cancer, or that all cancer patients are emotionally repressed! It simply indicates that having a repressed style is one of probably many factors—psychological, social and biological—that make cancer more likely to appear, and perhaps progress more rapidly.

It is worthwhile to take a closer look at some of the psychological factors whose possible impact on cancer have been studied. Stress of various kinds, including bereavement and other losses, is a factor that many patients cite as possible "causes" for their own cancer. Animal studies lend some support to this theory: it is possible to set up experiments with lab animals in a very controlled, consistent way, and to show that under certain conditions, a stress will reliably promote cancer growth. For example, in a fascinating series of experiments, Lawrence Sklar and Hymie Anisman showed that in mice with tumours who received an electric shock, those animals who were able to escape from the shock had slower tumour growth than control mice who received exactly the same shock but had no control over it![3] We have to be cautious in extrapolating from mice to people, but this discovery at least points to the possible value of having some personal control over one's environment. Human stress studies have given frustratingly variable results, however. One of the first was by Lawrence LeShan (cited in chapter 1 as a pioneer in the field), in 1956. He interviewed several hundred people, some with cancer and some without, and found that the cancer patients were much more likely to report severe life stressors in the years immediately preceding the interview. This would not now be acceptable as evidence (although it was standard for the time), mainly on the grounds that other differences between the patients and non-patients may have explained the different results, or that having cancer led to a difference in retrospective recall of life events. Many contrary results have been reported since. A prospective (looking-forward) investigation would obviously be more reliable—but this would seem to require assessing stress in thousands of people in order to find a small number, perhaps a few dozen, who developed cancer over some manageable period of time, say the next 5 to 10 years.

This latter kind of investigation has in fact been done to test the association between clinical depression and subsequently developing cancer. Depression is one of the qualities often measured in surveys of the health of large numbers of people for other reasons. In studies of this kind, scientists can follow people for many years, and relate the appearance of cancer, or other disease, to earlier mental qualities. An early investigation appeared to show that depressed individuals were more at risk[4]—but several large, later experiments contradicted this finding.[5]

Social support—for example, being married—is, however, a consistent protective factor against dying from many causes, and it appears to help in cancer as well. Here we do meet a difficulty of interpretation that we have already discussed, when distinguishing effects of the mind that act directly or "internally" on cancer, and others that might act indirectly or "externally" (chapter 1). It is difficult to know whether having good support means that one's physical needs are better cared for, or whether it is the conviction that others care that translates into a healthier state of mind and body that opposes cancer growth more effectively. One well-known study that seems to support the latter pathway was done by Bedell-Thomas and associates, who in 1946 gave a number of questionnaires to medical students, then followed them for up to 40 years (!) to see who developed various disease conditions. Subjects contracting cancer reported lack of closeness to parents at the early phase of life.[6] This is an extremely interesting point, but a skeptic could reasonably say that this early lack of support translated into later difficulties in forming close relationships, and hence poorer physical care in later life! Personally, I think it much more likely that distance from important family members while growing up generates a way of coping in the world that substantially affects one's physiology.

This latter interpretation is supported by the work of a brilliant researcher, Lydia Temoshok, who has developed a comprehensive, evidence-based theory linking early life events, subsequent adaptive style, and the risk of later cancer.[7] Temoshok was working in the late 1970s with people who had malignant melanoma (a dangerous skin cancer), and was struck by their unusual tendency to repress expression of emotions. In a series of experiments she demonstrated a correlation between such repression and higher risk for development or faster growth of cancer. Her interviews showed that this appeared to be a lifelong way of coping. Temoshok described a "Type C" personality, or as she prefers to call it, adaptive style, which is different in almost every way from the well-known hard-driving, hostile, impatient Type A personality believed to be associated with heart disease (chapter 2). Type C's (as described in the book by Temoshok and Dreher, *The Type C Connection*), are unassertive, patient, appeasing, often unaware of any "negative" emotions, particularly anger, not likely to experience or express anxiety, fear, or sadness, and tending to be overly concerned with meeting the needs of others, to the neglect of their own. The perceptive reader may begin to see a familiar pattern here: these people are living "inauthentic" lives, opposite to the free expression and permission to live as desired that we found to be characteristic of remarkable survivors. Temoshok hypothesized that the Type C style developed early in life as a way of coping with powerful figures like parents (recall Bedell-Thomas's medical students). She found that a crisis like cancer could lead, in these people, to one of three broad kinds of response: the path of transformation, or change to a more expressive (authentic) way of being; to entrenchment or maintaining the style, often more fiercely than before; or to resignation, giving up in hopelessness. These differing responses were shown to correlate in the expected way, not with lifespan in these early studies, but to differing seriousness of disease. Earlier investigations had indicated a relationship of repression to more severe disease, and there have been more since, so her ideas are consistent with findings of others; as I said, this is one area in which some general agreement can be found, although few in the field have paid Temoshok's hypothesis the attention it deserves.

The hopelessness aspect of the theory has also been borne out in other work: the idea that if a person learns early that she has no right to assert her needs, then a crisis like cancer will often cause a general giving up. This had previously been noted in connection with tendency to other psychosomatic (mind–body) disease. In the cancer field, Steven Greer, a psychiatrist working in London in the mid 1970s, interviewed women who recently underwent a mastectomy as treatment for primary cancer. He found that those patients who displayed a "fighting spirit," or who tended to minimize the seriousness of the disease, were significantly more likely to be alive 15 years later than others in the study who reacted with "stoic acceptance" or helplessness/hopelessness.[8] These last two kinds of response seem to be an aspect of the Type C pattern.

WHY HAS RESEARCH ON PERSONALITY AND CANCER PRODUCED SO LITTLE CONSENSUS?

The case for adjusting psychological state as part of the regular treatment of cancer would be greatly strengthened if researchers could agree on psychological factors that affect the disease. Although the data suggest that repression of emotions, hopelessness, and lack of social support may increase the risk of getting cancer and allow faster progression, results are not consistent or strong enough to be convincing to a skeptical person. For anyone who wishes to argue, as I do, that care of the patient's mind may be relevant to the course of his or her disease, it is important to account for negative or inconsistent results like these. I will point out here some of the reasons why many of the experiments carried out in the "personality–cancer" field are, in fact, poorly suited to uncovering a relationship. A more potent way of investigating the question (using psychological therapies to modify lifespan) will be discussed in the next section.

The first obstacle to demonstrating that one's state of mind might influence the progression of cancer derives from the particular scientific approach now in vogue. An excellent example is a study carried out by a first-rate researcher, Maggie Watson, who was also a colleague of Greer's.[9] Watson and colleagues gave a series of questionnaires to 578 women with early-stage breast cancer, and then noted their survival over at least 5 years. They found that women scoring high on helplessness and hopelessness had a small but significantly greater tendency than others to die during this time. "Fighting spirit" had no apparent effect on survival, in contradiction to the results of the earlier Greer report.

This type of study is currently most admired in the field, and indeed across much of the social sciences. The large number of women, the rigorous design, the cautious presentation and discussion of conclusions, even, perhaps, the finding that "fighting spirit" was not important to survival, allowed the acceptance of the paper by a top medical journal (*Lancet*). In their discussion, the authors suggested that "women can be relieved of the burden of guilt that occurs when they find it difficult to maintain a fighting spirit," a conclusion that was picked up by prominent news media. (Obviously this also implies that there is no clinical rationale for encouraging people to "fight" the disease, which flies in the face of much clinical experience and common sense). Yet when one looks closely at the paper, it really tells us very little about what does or does not help people live longer. Participants were asked to register their "fighting spirit" by endorsing items like "I keep quite busy, so I don't have time to think about it," "I count my blessings," as well as others that seem more germane like "I try to fight the illness." This kind of casual self-report can give only a very superficial impression of what people were really thinking. Subjects will often provide invalid responses, either because they want to be socially acceptable, or because their defensiveness prevents them from recognizing what they really feel (Type C individuals are especially prone to this tendency). By contrast, the earlier Greer study, which did show benefits to fighting spirit, incorporated one-to-one interviews with its subjects. Any clinician knows that skilled interviewing, although not infallible, can give a much more valid picture of what an individual is really thinking and feeling. Nevertheless, the usual practice in much of health psychology, including psycho-oncology, is to avoid the time-consuming work of interviewing patients and to rely instead on superficial self-report data, obtained at a single point in time, and readily translatable into impressive statistics. I have done this myself, for many years, but my later experience with the kind of detailed note taking and interviewing of patients over a period of time (chapters 5 and 6) has convinced me that this more hands-on approach is necessary if we truly want to understand how psychological factors are influencing health.

A second limitation of the Watson study, common to most in the area, is that the assessment was done at only one point in time. People's moods may, of course, vary widely from one day to the next. To uncover habitual attitudes to life, we need to hear from individuals on a number of occasions; we need to get to know them. Again, this is an expensive approach, in terms of professional time and research money, although all would agree that repeated contacts provide a more reliable estimate. Thus in both the method of assessment commonly used, and the frequency with which it is done, the norm is to favour inexpensive but superficial methods, allowing the use of a larger number of subjects, over more in-depth and repeated analyses with relatively few subjects. Although the Greer study, using interviews, had one-tenth the number of subjects of the Watson study, it is much more likely, I believe, to be uncovering valid relationships between psychology and disease progression.

A third reason why experiments relating psychological properties to survival in cancer patients are unlikely to demonstrate a relationship is perhaps the most important of all, yet it has been almost universally ignored in this literature. To understand it we need to consider the biology of cancer. When a tumour is found, it has already been growing for months or even years, as was pointed out in chapter 2. The cells comprising it have been subject to constant selection—only those that find the internal environment of the host person tolerable will have survived. This internal environment has been influenced by many factors, among them the psychological makeup of the host person. So the cancer has, as it were, learned to grow in that person, regardless of whether he or she is repressed or not, whether she has a fighting spirit or not, how emotionally close she is to other people, and so on. Thus assessments made at a single point in time are not only unreliable, as already argued, but also largely irrelevant, once a cancer has adapted to its host: whatever the person's psychological profile, his cancer is accustomed to it, and will continue to grow in it. For the mind to influence an established cancer, there

75

must logically be mental *change*, and change sufficient to affect the molecules that ultimately regulate cancer growth—acting through the long-range (neuro-endocrine) and short-range messenger pathways that we alluded to in chapter 2. Very few experiments indeed have attempted to look at such change (which is again more demanding than single-point assessment). This point cogently suggests that our best chance of describing an impact of mind on cancer progression will be in studies where a therapy is introduced to promote psychological change. We turn now to such experiments.

TESTING THE EFFECTS OF PSYCHOLOGICAL THERAPIES ON LIFESPAN

If we accept the logical necessity for change if the mind is to affect cancer progression, then the most direct way to test it would be to see whether a psychological therapy, designed to induce change, can prolong survival. We have seen in chapter 3 that "remarkable survivors" tend to say that they have changed considerably as a reaction to their diagnosis, but we have also discussed how difficult it is to rely on this kind of subjective self-report. Investigators have begun to test the possible impact of psychological interventions on lifespan in cancer patients. This is still a very new endeavour, since it is only recently that the possibility of life extension through such therapy has been taken at all seriously by people equipped to test it.

The credit for this interest belongs mainly to a Stanford psychiatrist, David Spiegel. Spiegel trained with a renowned psychotherapist, Irvin Yalom, in the 1970s, and in collaboration with him and other colleagues, showed that support groups for women with metastatic breast cancer were not, as had been feared, frightening and possibly harmful to participants, but were in fact very useful in helping them cope with the distress caused by their situation. This was already a pioneering finding, which helped secure the current acceptance of such groups. These experiments were designed to test only relatively short-term effects on quality of life. However, in 1989, some 10 years later, Spiegel took the further step of examining the survival data on the people from the earlier experiments. To his apparent surprise, he and his colleagues found that women who had been in a support group for a year or more had lived approximately twice as long after their diagnosis as similar women who had not been in the therapy.[10] This result created a quite a stir in New Age and other circles! It appeared to confirm what many had hoped—the power of the mind to influence the course of a serious disease. Now, 14 years later, and after a number of similar experiments, the picture is less clear. At the time of writing there are 11 such trials published, to my knowledge, 5 giving positive results (some prolongation of life) and 6 with negative results. To understand this ambiguity we need to examine the methods used in these studies.

The currently preferred way to test the therapeutic value of any agent or procedure, whether a drug or a psychological approach, is to enter subjects into a randomized controlled trial. The "controlled" part means that some of the patients get the intervention, while others do not, so that a comparison of outcomes can be made. "Randomizing" means that subjects are assigned to either intervention or control on a random or chance basis. This is the best method we have of ensuring that other factors (variables) which, although unrecognized, might have an important influence on outcome, are on average similar in the 2 groups. Most of the published trials have used randomization; a minority have assigned patients to the two comparison groups in other ways. This technology was developed by the eminent statistician R. A. Fisher early in the last century, as a way of testing the effect of fertilizers on agricultural plots, and it has been widely adopted to test the effectiveness of drugs in medical research. Essentially it works well for drug research, but there are important limitations in applying it to testing the effects of a psychological therapy.

The principal limiting factor in using randomized controlled trials (RCTs) to test whether or not psychological therapies prolong life is that subjects are lumped into 2 large groups: those who get the intervention, and those who do not. The experimenter then plots, on a graph, the rate at which subjects die in each group. In essence, averages or median survival times are calculated for each group. The experiment tests only whether or not the survival of the group as a whole is enhanced by the therapy. It is not very sensitive to effects of the therapy on a small minority; if a minority do something unusual, and enhance their survival, it would usually be lost in the comparison of group means. For example, in an experiment in which 100 cancer patients received an intervention, and 100 did not, if 10 of the intervention subjects made the kinds of personal transformation that the "remarkable survivors" of chapter 3 report, and lived twice as long as expected, this fact would in most cases be undetectable statistically in an RCT. This problem is much more important in assessing psychotherapies than in testing drugs, because the variability in the way people react to or make use of psychotherapy is much greater than the variability in response to drugs. Provided a drug is taken, one can be reasonably sure that it will have a certain definable physiological effect. But attendance at psychotherapy sessions provides no such guarantee. In fact, many of those attending make no use of the therapy at all, while others may transform their lives. Thus the very subjects of most interest to those of us looking for a potential effect of psychological change on survival may be hidden behind a majority of "non-compliers." A study with a relatively large percentage of people who made good use of the intervention might score "positive," while one in which most did not would likely be "negative."

A related problem is that, not surprisingly, people don't like to be randomly assigned to one group or another—they prefer to choose. So, many individuals with cancer refuse to enter studies like these. It is likely that among those refusing are the people most determined to help themselves. Even worse, from the point of view of the investigators, they might join the study but if assigned to the control group, venture out and find an alternative source of the intervention elsewhere (this happens a lot—it goes by the technical name of "contamination"!).

A third limitation of studies in this area so far has been that the interventions used have not been designed to induce profound psychological change. They have also been highly variable in nature, ranging from 6 weekly sessions of "behavioural therapy" to a year of weekly group supportive discussions. This variation has contributed, no doubt, to the variety in results obtained. Most important, to reiterate what has been pointed out already, for a valid test of the impact of mind, the psychological change must be sufficient to alter the internal regulators of cancer growth (chapter 2) if we are to expect an effect on lifespan.

Perhaps the most inoffensive way to illustrate how these problems affect results is to show an experiment conducted by our own group and published in 1998 (Figure 4.1). This was an RCT designed specifically to test whether an intervention could prolong life in cancer patients (most prior results, like Spiegel's, were retrospective analyses, performed as an afterthought, which for technical reasons diminishes their credibility). The subjects involved in our study were women with medically incurable metastatic breast cancers. They did not, as a rule, seek out the intervention, but were identified from the hospital clinic records and asked to participate; thus they were not particularly highly motivated. The intervention was basically a supportive one, with some training in coping skills, provided by a skilled group therapist. Subjects attended a weekly group for one year. Most did very little healing work at home (again indicating little real motivation for change—see chapter 5). As the figure shows, there may have been a slight tendency for those in the intervention to do better than the controls, but this was not statistically significant. Subsequently there has been a much larger, similar experiment by Goodwin and colleagues[11] with the same result.

We were, of course, disappointed with our result—the experiment was an attempt to replicate Spiegel's encouraging finding, as was Goodwin's. In other published trials where a positive effect has been found, the size of this effect has been small. The 3 technically most reliable RCTs designed specifically to test life extension (ours, Goodwin's, and another by Edelman and colleagues in 1999), have all yielded negative results. In retrospect, this finding is perhaps not surprising, given the limitations of this experimental approach that I have noted above. The consensus now is that interventions

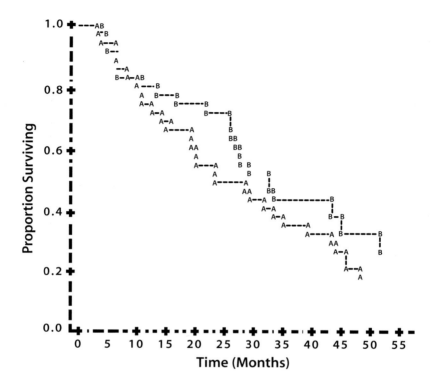

FIGURE 4.1 *A cumulative plot of the number of women surviving at different times after enrolling in the randomized controlled study conducted by Cunningham et al. (1998). The group receiving the intervention is shown as "B," and the controls as "A." (Reproduced with permission from John Wiley and Sons Ltd.)*

of this kind do not increase *average* survival among such patients. Unfortunately, this has been taken, in some quarters, to indicate that the issue is closed—that psychological help and change generally can prolong life for no cancer patients, and that the mind cannot affect cancer progression. While many scientifically oriented physicians and some psychologists would, perhaps unthinkingly, draw this negative conclusion at present, I hope it is clear that such a sweeping generalization would be unjustified on the evidence. We can only say, from these trials, that *therapy of the types employed* appears to have no significant *average* effect on the lifespan of the particular (usually not highly motivated) patients tested.

In common with most who do relatively intensive and long-term psychological therapy with cancer patients, I was unhappy with the state of play resulting from the clinical trials approach, including the results of our own study. It seemed obvious to me that some patients, particularly those who got strongly involved in trying to help themselves psychologically and spiritually, lived much longer than expected. Other therapists to whom I have spoken about this have generally agreed. Perhaps we were missing these people in our trials, "losing" their good survivals in the calculated averages? How could they be identified among a majority of less involved people?

This problem, of course, is not new, and has been addressed by many scientists trying to assess the outcomes of psychotherapies of various kinds. Instead of comparing group means we may need to look at what patients do *individually*, and relate each person's efforts to his or her ultimate survival. This may seem like common sense—it is the kind of assessment we make in ordinary life, after all—but it is a strategy that has been largely disregarded in medical science. A person highly involved in self-healing might tend to live much longer, other things being equal, than another individual not so involved. It is an approach that is essential, I would argue, if we are going to understand how to help people live longer in the face of serious disease. We must study first those who make an all-out effort, learn from them, and then apply what we have learned to help others who do not currently get very involved, but might well do so if they were assured of a path that could bring results for them. The conclusions reached by people like LeShan and the Simontons (chapter 1) were based on this kind of observation, although they did not have a reliable way of determining whether individuals had outlived their life expectancies. Is it possible to do a rigorous, prospective, experiment of this type? In the next chapter I will describe our efforts in this direction.

SUMMARY

After describing some of the questions addressed by the new discipline of "psycho-oncology," including its focus on how cancer influences mental state, I moved to a discussion of research on the reverse effect, how the mind may affect onset and progression of cancer. There is an enormous and undoubted impact of unhealthy behaviours, such as smoking and aspects of diet, on incidence of cancer. Of more relevance to us here, however, is the possible impact of mental change on progression of existing cancers by some "internal" pathway, that is, by affecting the inner state of the body in such a way as to oppose the growth of a cancer.

The two main approaches to this question were discussed. The first comprises half a century of efforts to correlate aspects of "personality" or adaptive styles to the growth of cancer. Results have been inconsistent, although there is some consensus that repression of emotions makes development of cancer more likely, and that social support may impede its progression. We looked at some of the reasons why it may be difficult to detect a real effect using this kind of method. The second approach is experimental: can psychological therapies prolong life in cancer patients? Again, results have been mixed; of II published studies, 5 have given (mostly very small) positive effects, and 6, including those most technically reliable, have yielded negative findings. These studies were designed to look for overall impact on the average survival of participants; they were not designed to detect any impact on lifespan of an unusual degree of mental change in a minority of highly motivated patients. All also employed therapies that were basically supportive, rather than aiming at inducing change. However, the upshot of these inconsistent findings is that most health professionals would currently regard a potential therapeutic effect of mind on cancer as unproven and unlikely.

REFERENCES

1. Andersen, B. L., & gy. In A. M Nezu & C. M. Nezu (Eds.), *Handbook of psychology: Vol. 9. Health Psychology* (pp. 267–292). New York: John Wiley & Sons.
2. Dalton, S. O., Boesen, E. H., Ross, L., Shapiro, I. R., & Johansen, C. (2002). Mind and cancer: Do psychological factors cause cancer? *European Journal of Cancer, 38*(10), 1313–1323.

    Edelman, S., & Kidman, A. D. (1997). Mind and cancer: Is there a relationship? A review of evidence. *Australian Psychologist, 32*(2), 79–85.

    Fox, B. H. (1998). Psychosocial factors in cancer incidence and prognosis. In J. C. Holland (Ed.), *Psycho-Oncology* (pp. 110–124). New York: Oxford University.

    Kreitler, S., Chaitchik, S., & Kreitler, H. (1993). Repression: Cause or result of cancer? *Psycho-Oncology, 2*, 43–54.

    McKenna, M. C., Zevon, M. A., Corn, B., & Rounds, J. (1999). Psychosocial factors and the development of breast cancer: A meta-analysis. *Health Psychology, 18*, 520–531.
3. Sklar, L. S., & Anisman, H. (1979). Stress and coping factors influence tumor growth. *Science, 205*(4405), 513–515; Sklar, L. S., & Anisman, H. (1980). Social stress influences tumor growth. *Psychosomatic Medicine, 42*(3), 347–365.
4. Shekelle, R. B., Raynor, W. J., Ostfeld, A. M., Garron, D. C., Bieliauskas, L. A., Liu, S. C., et al. Psychological depression and 17-year risk of death from cancer. *Psychosomatic Medicine, 43*(2), 117–125.
5. Dalton, S. O., Mellemkjaer, L., Olsen, J. H., Mortensen, P. B., & Johansen, C. (2002). Depression and cancer risk: A register-based study of patients hospitalized with affective disorders, Denmark, 1969–1993. *American Journal of Epidemiology, 155*(12), 1088–1095.

    Fox, B. H. (1995). A hypothesis to reconcile conflicting conclusions in studies relating depressed mood to later cancer. In M. Stein & A. Baum (Eds.), *Chronic diseases*. Mahwah, NJ: Lawrence Erlbaum Associates.

    Mathe, G. (1996). Depression, stressful events and the risk of cancer (Editorial). *Biomedicine & Pharmacotherapy, 50*(1), 1–2.
6. Shaffer, J. W., Duszynski, K. R., & Thomas, C. B. (1982). Family attitudes in youth as a possible precursor of cancer among physicians: A search for explanatory mechanisms. *Journal of Behavioral Medicine, 5*(2), 143–163.

    Thomas, C. B. (1988). Cancer and the youthful mind: A forty-year perspective. *Advances, 5*(2), 42–58; Thomas, C. B., Duszynksi, K. R., & Shaffer, J. W. (1979). Family attitudes reported in youth as potential predictors of cancer. *Psychosomatic Medicine, 41*, 287–302.
7. Temoshok, L., & Dreher, H. (1992). *The Type C connection: The behavioral links to cancer and your health*. New York: Random House.

Temoshok, L. (2000). Complex coping patterns and their role in adaptation and neuroimmunomodulation: Theory, methodology, and research. *Annals of the New York Academy of Sciences, 917,* 446–455.

Temoshok, L. (2002). Connecting the dots linking mind, behavior, and disease: The biological concomitants of coping patterns: Commentary on "Attachment and cancer: A conceptual integration." *Integrative Cancer Therapies, 1*(4), 387-391.

8. Greer, S., Morris, T., & Pettingale, K. W. (1979). Psychological response to breast cancer: Effect on outcome. *Lancet, 2*(8146), 785–787.

   Greer, S., Morris, T., Pettingale, K. W., & Haybittle, J. (1990). Psychological response to breast cancer and 15-year outcome. *Lancet, 335*(8680), 49–50.

9. Watson, M., Haviland, J. S., Greer, S., Davidson, J., & Bliss, J. M. (1999). Influence of psychological response on survival in breast cancer: A population-based cohort study. *Lancet, 354,* 1331–1336.

10. Spiegel, D., Bloom, J., Kraemer, H. C., & Gottleib, E. (1989). Effect of psycho-social treatment on survival of patients with metastatic breast cancer. *Lancet, 2*(8668), 888–891.

11. Goodwin, P. J., Leszcz, M., Ennis, M., Koopmans, J., Vincent, L., Guther, H., et al. (2001). The effect of group psychosocial support on survival in metastatic breast cancer. *New England Journal of Medicine, 345*(24), 1719–1726.

Chapter 5

Working Towards Longer Survival: The Healing Journey Study

We come now to what has been the main stimulus for writing this book: a series of systematic clinical and research investigations that we have carried out over the last 10 years, on the kinds of psychological properties and change that appear to promote longer survival in people with serious cancers. The reader should be aware that this is very much a work in progress, and a minority view at present; no other group has yet undertaken the kind of rigorous, prospective experimental test of the qualities favouring survival that I will outline, and replication by others will be needed for the ideas to gain acceptance. I present them here because they mesh so well with clinical observations by ourselves and by a large number of other professionals, with the studies on remarkable survivors (chapter 3), and with the evidence on Type C adaptation and repression as a risk factor in cancer (chapter 4). When all of these results are put together, and notwithstanding the conflicting results from clinical trials presented in the last chapter, I believe we can sketch a plausible picture of the role the mind may play in assisting healing from cancer, and I will devote the rest of the book to discussing it. If we wait for certainty, we may wait a long time.

There are two main features of the experimental work I am going to describe that are unusual in the field of psycho-oncology, yet necessary to overcome the limitations of the more popular "randomized trials" approach that was discussed in the last chapter:

1. the development and use of a form of psychological therapy for cancer patients that can provide a structure to guide those people who are motivated to work towards substantial personal change

2. the use of a correlative design, rather than a comparison of group means, so that the efforts and changes made by each individual can be related to his or her life extension (explained below)

I will first describe our Healing Journey therapy program, which has been developed over the last 20 years. The basic aim of the program is to help patients cope better with their disease, and to improve the quality of their life. A secondary aim, often uppermost in the minds of those who have attended, is to prolong life. I'll then describe a completed experiment that strongly suggests an impact of dedicated psychological self-help work on survival in at least some people with medically incurable cancers. A replication of this experiment is currently underway. In the following chapter I will document interviews conducted with 10 people from our program many years after they had survived a medical prediction of early death, contrasting what they said with statements made by other cancer patients who failed to outlive their prognoses, and with members of a third group interviewed before entering a course of therapy.

A STEPWISE PROGRAM OF THERAPY: THE HEALING JOURNEY

While some people with cancer need individual psychiatric or psychotherapy treatments, the majority are psychologically healthy, but highly stressed by the diagnosis. As discussed in the last chapter, many can be greatly helped by meeting in groups with other cancer patients; such meetings diminish the sense of isolation, allow sharing of emotions (with peers who understand and can listen), and provide a venue for learning from others and solving problems, such as how best to relate to family, doctors, and friends. Groups are to be preferred for these reasons, and because they are obviously more economical than one-to-one consultations with health care professionals. They are also a convenient forum for learning and practising specific coping techniques; among those we teach are deep relaxation, various kinds of mental imaging and drawing, watching one's thoughts, setting goals, meditating, consulting a source of "inner wisdom," keeping a journal, reading appropriate books on healing and spirituality, and other methods.[1]

Our efforts to provide a group program for cancer patients and interested family members began in 1982. For some years, meetings were held mostly in private homes and in rooms generously made available by the Canadian Cancer Society, but in recent times most of the work has been done at the cancer hospital where I am employed. As we learned what helps most, we gradually refined the methods and ways of presenting them. It became evident fairly quickly that many people, on "graduating" from a basic course of what was then six to nine weekly sessions, wanted further support and more advanced instruction. We added a second level or stage to the program in 1985, and soon after followed that with a third, these two higher levels usually involving eight weekly meetings, in small (5–12 member) groups. The third level was, for many years, a process of writing one's "life story," and then presenting it to the rest of the group—an uplifting experience (once the initial trepidation was overcome!), and one that often clarified for the participant what the main themes of her life had been, and what was of top priority now. More recently, the third-level agenda has changed to eight sessions on spiritual aspects of healing. For the last 10 years or so, a limited number of patients with metastatic cancers have been enrolled in a fourth level, consisting of weekly therapy groups in which the emphasis has been on further psychological and spiritual growth. These more intensive and long-running groups, restricted to small numbers of patients because of our limited resources, have been the main source of information for the work on prolongation of life described below. Steps 1 to 3 thus constitute our "core" program, with Level 4 as an extra, for patients with terminal prognoses. Table 5.1 summarizes the content of the program in its current form.

At present, we enrol 200 to 300 new patients every year, with all kinds and stages of cancer. About half are accompanied by a family member to the Level 1 course (which is now shortened to four sessions, delivered in a small auditorium to groups of 50 or so, and repeated five or more times per year). About half of the patients in Level 1 elect to move on to Level 2; at this stage, smaller groups are used for at least part of the sessions, to allow sharing, and the family members have a separate group of their own. Most of these people proceed to Level 3: whether or not people continue through the program depends on many factors, in addition to their health and preferences—for example, availability of staff and rooms, and the vigour with which continuing is advocated!

Those wanting details on the content of the program, and the many research papers that have been written based on its work, can find information on our website www.healingjourney.ca, or in our papers cited in the references for this chapter. For the present, our focus will be on the properties of this kind of program that make it especially suited to investigating our main question: can mental change affect the progression of cancer?

The first thing to emphasize about the Healing Journey is its stepwise nature. This allows participants to try a short exposure in Level 1, then either proceed to the next step, or drop out if they have had as much help as they want. Remarkably, this kind of structure is still virtually unknown in psycho-oncology (although used in other areas, like addiction counselling). Almost all other therapies in common use are single stage, and typically of 6 to 12 weeks' duration (although some, as in the Spiegel study cited earlier, involve a year or more of group support for a small number of patients). For research purposes, the stepped structure acts as a kind of filter, concentrating, so to speak, the people who wish to become most engaged with the work.

A second point about the Healing Journey is that it presents self-healing as a *learning* process. Support is valued, but seen as not enough

TABLE 5.1 *Main Elements of the Healing Journey Program*

Level 1: Taking Control: Coping with Cancer Stress (four sessions)
- Communicating feelings
- Deep relaxation
- Thought monitoring and changing
- Mental imagery
- Setting goals

Level 2: Getting Connected: Skills for Healing (eight sessions)
- Journalling (self-examination)
- Consulting "inner wisdom": the "Inner Healer" technique
- Meditation: mind quieting
- Dropping resentments
- Setting goals

Level 3: Finding Meaning: Steps to Spiritual Healing (eight sessions)
- Understanding spirituality
- Identifying and dropping the obstacles to spiritual connection
- Spiritual practices (meditation, prayer, chanting, reading, meeting with others)

Level 4: Long-term group therapy (psychological and spiritual content)
- Discussion group for graduates of Levels 3 and 4 (ongoing)

---

if the participant wishes to gain some control over his or her experience. Appropriate and effective techniques, like those I listed above, can be learned and practised. As a simple example, someone who constantly wakes through the night with anxious thoughts may be greatly helped by knowing how to "watch" her mind, counter some of the frightening thoughts, and use a relaxation technique to get back to sleep. A more sophisticated example is the "Inner Healer" imagery method in which people learn to contact a previously unrecognized source of wisdom within themselves, personified as a spiritual or ancestral figure who can often provide answers to troubling questions.

A third feature of the program is its emphasis, in the later stages, on spirituality and healing. Spiritual or existential concerns are absolutely central in the minds of many cancer patients ("Is this the end? Is there a God, and if so, why did this happen to me?"), and some answers may come through meditation, prayer, or spiritual discussion and reflection. Figure 5.1 arranges various techniques and therapeutic approaches as a hierarchy, becoming more demanding as one ascends, but also potentially more life-transforming. It is emphasized that no guarantees can be offered for effects on the physical disease, only that work of this kind will improve quality of life and *may* have an effect on progression, depending on many factors, including the nature of the cancer itself. Thus there is no cause for blaming oneself if the cancer continues to grow at the same rate in the face of one's best efforts.

While our program attempts to help people progress through various stages of healing, we would certainly not claim that our program is the only or even necessarily the best way to do so; the structure we present is simply one form, adapted over the years to the people seeking help from us, of a fairly widely understood process of psychological and spiritual growth. We have ample documentation of its ability to improve quality of life; for the purpose of investigating possible extension of life, it will be seen that it provides us with a way to both select and encourage motivated cancer patients, a kind of framework for personal evolution. The keenest participants typically seek out additional things to do to help themselves at other locations, and are encouraged to do so (something we took into account in the study described below).

Before moving to a discussion of research design, I would like here to acknowledge the collaboration of many dedicated health

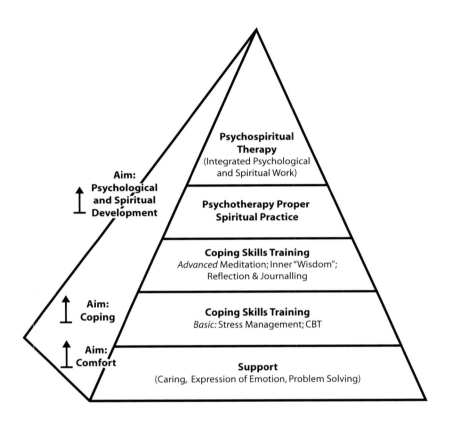

FIGURE 5.1 *Types of psychological therapy, arranged in order of increasing demands made on the participant as the pyramid is ascended. CBT = cognitive behavioural therapy. (Reproduced from A.J. Cunningham (2002), Group psychological therapy: An integral part of care for cancer patients,* Integrative Cancer Therapies, 1, 67-75, *with permission, Sage Publications Inc.)*

professionals in the operation of this program over the last 15 years of its existence. Claire Edmonds and Cathy Phillips, both initially graduate students in my team and now with doctoral degrees in psychology, have been superb therapists and researchers. Many other professionals have either observed the program or contributed (by leading small groups) over this time. Among our devoted course co-ordinators (front-line workers who staff the phones and try to help people who call in great distress) have been Heather Hanson, Gwen Jenkins, Nancy Folk, and Jan Ferguson. Gina Lockwood has been a valued statistical consultant over the years, and David Hedley has been prominent among the medical staff who have assisted us.

A RESEARCH DESIGN TO SEARCH FOR EFFECTS OF MIND ON LONGEVITY

Armed with an ongoing therapy program that seems clinically to encourage substantial psychological change in at least some partici-pants, and brings to the fore a steady stream of people with an in-terest in self-healing, how might we best design an experiment to test our question? Simply observing the patients passing through a program and forming an impression is obviously not enough—we are all too prone to seeing what we want to believe. For a rigorous study, certain requirements must be satisfied. The study should ideally be prospective and longitudinal, technical terms meaning that we want to enrol patients, make some prediction of their likely survival, and follow them over time to see how well they do, as opposed to identi-fying survivors long after their experience and asking them what they did in the past (as in the studies of chapter 3). To obtain an indication of the impact of self-help on survival, we need first to get the best possible expert prediction of likely survival duration, and then com-pare it with actual survival time. As a result we will be able to say, for example, this person survived 2, 3, or 5 times longer than medically predicted. The therapy needs to be as intense as we can make it. And finally, we need a comprehensive characterization of the psychologi-cal state of participants, to identify those qualities that are associated with longer survival.

Details of our experiment can be found in our published papers[2] and on our website.[3] In brief, our first experiment of this kind involved 22 patients with medically incurable cancers (the types most commonly represented were metastatic breast cancer, metastatic colo-rectal cancer, and pancreatic cancer). These people entered the Healing Journey therapy groups for a year (a few dropped out before the year was over). Relevant data from the medical charts for each patient at the time of entry were examined independently by between 9 and 14 oncologists at the Princess Margaret Hospital; each expert made a prediction of likely lifespan, and a median (mid-range) estimate was calculated. Psychological descriptions were made from analysis of verbal "data," meaning regular written homework assignments and therapists' notes, which were collected each week for each participant (sometimes 100 pages or more in total). These data were subjected to a standard process called qualitative analysis, from which a large number of themes was derived, themes like "dedication to self-help work" or "awareness of the changes needed."

The qualitative analysis was done using special computer software that facilitated the clustering of each piece of verbal text under appropriate thematic headings (called "coding"). Thus all the material illustrating each theme could be swiftly drawn together. We then had to relate the strength of expression of each of these themes to survival, and for this purpose, numbers had to be assigned to them. Each of four psychologically trained raters inspected a summary of the data for each theme and provided a rating estimate, on a scale of 1 to 5. For example, under "dedication to self-help work," a rating of 1 indicated that there was little or no dedication displayed, and 5 meant that the person largely devoted his or her life to the healing work. The team debated (often vigorously!) what the final rating should be for each theme. To give the lay reader some idea of the exhaustive thoroughness of this analysis, coding the data for one subject might take 2 or more person-days. Inspecting it and deciding on a rating was a little easier: perhaps up to 1 day per subject, for each of the raters. Discussing and finalizing the rating for some 26 sub-themes—a day per subject. In addition was a lot of clerical work in arranging material, writing and refining scenarios to illustrate the scores of 1 to 5 on each theme. Thus the whole process took many thousands of person-hours of work. This contrasts with the relative ease of obtaining psychometric data (from self-report questionnaires) of the kind described in the last chapter, but having used both methods I can state that there is no comparison between the confidence one has in the conclusions. In fact, we used some standard self-report questionnaires as well, the scores on which failed to correlate with survival. We came to know our subjects intimately, and the team rating process assured a degree of objectivity. As a later refinement, we have had "blind" raters, who did not know the patients, examine an edited version of the data from which all mention of health matters, and all therapists' inferences, had been removed, in order to counter the possibility that we, the therapists, might have known from physical clues how long a person might be expected to survive.

Before looking at the results, I want to emphasize some of the differences between this study and the investigations that we have previously discussed. It differs from studies of "remarkable survivors" in several ways, most critically in being *prospective*. Rather than starting with known survivors, without having any idea how many others like them had not survived (chapter 3), we enrolled eligible people as they presented themselves, and followed all of them, noting survival for each. Another important point of difference is the care taken to obtain the best possible estimate of likely survival time for each patient, in contrast with the remarkable survivor studies where there were only retrospective and superficial estimates of likely survival. Note that we did not set up the experiment to detect only "cures" or "spontaneous remissions" (although we saw two of these). Instead, we focused on prolongation of lifespan beyond that expected, assisted by the stepwise therapy program. Under these conditions, it becomes possible to detect relatively modest effects, such as prolongation of life by a year or so (and see Figure 5.3). As discussed in chapter 3, cases of complete remissions of disease, especially where there has been no psychological help, are likely to be quite rare, so a prospective experiment that will detect nothing less than this is almost certain to fail.

Experiments using an RCT (controlled trials) design are currently regarded more highly in medical research, as I have said, because at least in principle they allow us to be more certain that an intervention *causes* an effect (in practice, this often is not the case—note the ambiguity surrounding results of trials in this area, as discussed in the last chapter). By contrast, if we find that a certain set of psychological qualities is associated with longer survival, we cannot formally conclude that these qualities caused the longer life, although, as we will see, it may be the most probable explanation. However, to reiterate, a correlative experiment like ours has the distinct advantage that the "performance" (survival beyond that predicted) for each person can be related to the psychological qualities he or she displayed. Because a small number of people were studied minutely, rather than a large number en masse, we obtained a detailed picture of what each individual did, and thus added to our knowledge about self-healing (there is no such learning in a trial, which is intended only to confirm or deny an effect of a therapy on an outcome). We were able to define a "dose–response" relationship between the qualities we were interested in and the outcome; in this case, survival. And we did not have to assign anyone randomly to a control group, which is a most unpleasant procedure, unacceptable to many of the patients, but instead were able to do the experiment under "real life" clinical conditions.

Almost all decisions in everyday life are made from correlations, which is also the way we accumulate clinical experience and indeed most medical knowledge. Unfortunately, there is a current fashion in medical research to look down upon correlative evidence, which diminishes the attention some health care professionals are willing to pay to findings from experiments like this.

RESULTS OF THE HEALING JOURNEY LONGEVITY STUDY

From the qualitative analysis of what participants wrote in their homework over a year, and notes taken by the group therapists at each weekly session, we developed a "model" or map of the process of changing in response to the threat to life, which agrees quite well with other research in the area of personal change, and is also a picture that makes sense. The model is shown in Figure 5.2. Each box encloses a major theme, which in turn comprises a number of sub-themes (not shown in the diagram). Thus people's "appraisal of threat" includes their perception of the need to change, awareness of what specifically they might do about it, and other sub-themes. The efforts that individuals make depend on this appraisal; then, given an awareness that change was necessary, the next step is the degree of willingness to actually do something, a theme that includes as sub-themes the abilities they think they have, and the outcomes they expect from their efforts. "Downstream" from this was the work actually done, and the dedication with which it is embraced: it is quite possible for someone to believe that work and change are needed, yet to lack motivation, or to have the motivation and not translate that into action for various reasons (such as lack of support at home). And influencing everything in this pathway is "ability to act and change," an assessment of pre-existing qualities in each person that to varying degrees paved the way to action or, in some cases, effectively prevented the individual from accomplishing much (examples of the latter would be a strong sense of inferiority or inadequacy, or a world view that was rather concrete and did not allow for mind–body effects). Ill health at the time of joining the study was not a factor that prevented the self-help work; all those enrolled had to be able to function relatively normally, although of course some had symptoms, like pain or weight loss as a result of their illness. All received standard medical care during the time with us, and that was taken into account by the oncologists in making their estimates of likely survival.

Dedicated application of self-help work (practice of the techniques taught, coupled with reflection and efforts to change), brought about a substantial improvement in what we called "quality of experience" (Figure 5.2). But did it prolong survival? There were various ways of testing this. One was to relate each theme to survival, using a technique called regression analysis, which basically means plot-

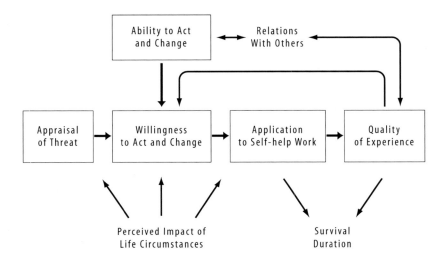

FIGURE 5.2 *A model of the psychological response to cancer, derived from the qualitative analysis of the Healing Journey study described in the text. (From Cunningham, Phillips, Stephen, and Edmonds, 2002. Reproduced with permission from Sage Publications Inc.)*

ting survival duration and the theme scores on a graph, and seeing how close the results are to a theoretical line representing a perfect relationship. All the major themes except "Appraisal" correlated significantly with survival. This remained the case when the individual health status of each subject was taken into account; in effect, we were then plotting psychological theme scores against the extent to which individuals outlived their medically predicted survival.

Regression analysis is a bit technical (the results obtained with it are described in our papers, referred to in the references to this chapter for those who want them). I will present a simpler way of looking at the outcome here. We added the scores for all the themes in the boxes in Figure 5.2 except for "quality of experience" and called this comprehensive score a measure of "involvement in self-help." We could then write down these scores, in rank order, for all 22 subjects.

We divided this list into thirds, representing "high," "medium," and "low" involvement respectively. We could now plot on a graph the median survival for each of these three subgroups against their survival (Figure 5.3).

The results were highly significant statistically, and really quite dramatic for work of this kind (p = 0.006 on the graph means that one could expect a result as strong as this by chance only once in about 200 repeat attempts). As you can see from the right-hand panel on the graph, the "high" involved subgroup, that is, the top 8 in terms of involvement, lived for a median time of nearly 3 years, and 2 of these people have had complete remissions of (supposedly fatal) disease for about 10 years now. By contrast, the "low" subgroup died at 1 year. The "medium" subgroup survived for an intermediate length of time. Was this difference caused by differences in their degree of illness? We can be fairly sure that it was not, for two main reasons. First, the left panel of the graph shows the median medical estimates of survival for all three subgroups at the time of entering the study: these were identical; in other words, people who *later* demonstrated low involvement were no sicker, on average, than those who later became highly involved. Second, the attendance at therapy sessions, a fair measure of health status, was not significantly different for the three subgroups; it was not the case that the "low involved" people suddenly became ill after joining the study—they were simply less enthusiastic from the start.

The most likely explanation for the results is that involvement in self-help promotes longer survival. Technically speaking, it is possible that some unidentified factor other than involvement was responsible for it, but nobody has been able to say what this might plausibly be. We would not wish to conclude that the therapy "caused" the longer survival, but rather that a combination of the personal qualities of the subjects, encouraged by the therapy, was probably responsible for it. Without the therapy, however, such large effects are unlikely, given the history of small and inconsistent results uncovered by the cross-sectional analyses I described in the last chapter.

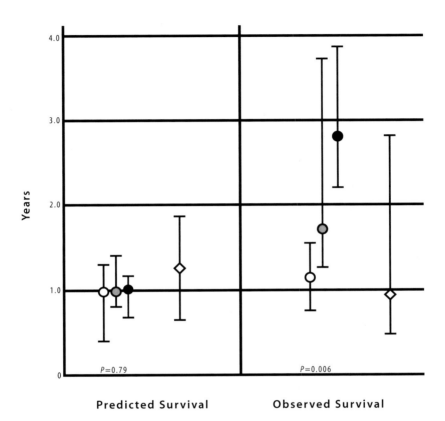

FIGURE 5.3 *The impact of "involvement in self-help" on survival. The left-hand panel shows the survival predicted by a panel of oncologists for the 3 subgroups of patients, with "low," "medium," and "high" involvement. The right-hand panel shows the actual survival of patients in these 3 categories. The diamond-shaped dots show that in a control group of 18 similar patients, the median survival predicted by the oncologists (left-hand panel) was similar to what was actually observed (right-hand panel). (From Cunningham, Phillips, Lockwood, Hedley, and Edmonds, 2000. Reproduced with permission, Innovision Communications.)*

ILLUSTRATING THE DIFFERING
"INVOLVEMENT" OF PARTICIPANTS

Let us look now in a more descriptive way at some of the contrasting qualities of people who were "high," "medium," or "low" in their involvement with self-help work.[4] The process of ranking the 22 patients allowed us to see a number of clusters of similar attitudes, members of the same cluster generally being adjacent to one another, or nearly so. (Note that in this clinical description we classed 9 as "highly involved," because of the similarities they displayed in their behaviours, 5 as "moderately," and 8, the lowest, as "low.")

Highly Involved People

Nine of the 22 subjects could be said to have been "highly involved" (the dividing lines between high, medium, and low were, of course, not sharp). These participants all developed a program for themselves that incorporated substantial changes in lifestyle, and included regular relaxation, imagery and thought monitoring, and a meditative or other spiritual practice. They were open to exploring new ways of thinking and behaving, and were disciplined in their work. Obstacles that they faced—demanding medical treatments, pain, deteriorating health status, family and work demands—were not allowed to interfere substantially with their personal program. All of these participants appeared to use what they learned from the therapy as a means of changing their lives.

The four persons ranked highest in their involvement stood out because they immersed themselves fully in the work, without reservation (we called them "wholeheartedly involved"). They found the psychological and spiritual exploration of compelling interest for its own sake, not simply as a means to a possible cure. They also initiated and explored self-help activities beyond those offered in the program.

Examples:

> *"I find self-exploration really exciting . . . There is true joy in this process along with the challenges. I welcome the challenge, as this is where the change takes place."*

> *"I do my relaxation exercises prior to my meditation/prayer/ imaging sessions, which I do about 9:30 each a.m. As well, I do relaxation each afternoon before a (shorter) meditation and a nap . . . I am trying to add additional meditation and visualization sessions in the late afternoon and in the evening, which are preceded by relaxation. I have also started doing a tai chi routine at various intervals during the day."*

> *"I spend up to 2 hours a day in meditation, prayer, visualization, and spiritual reading; most days. If I miss mornings, I do some at night."*

> *"I am working through the Course in Miracles workbook [a modern spiritual text], which is giving me a tremendous dose of spiritual- ity. . . . I meditate for 20 minutes every morning on the lesson for the day, and think about it when I can during the day. I lose my awareness of time when I meditate on these phrases; they feel like they are being poured inside of me."*

Effort of this kind brought substantial rewards. All of the people at the top end of the involvement scale enjoyed relatively good quality of life experience. An example:

> *"Spiritual oneness stays with me. Anything that isn't done with love feels like an insult to everything. I have deep feelings of rever- ence. Right now I feel better than ever in my life."*

Unlike the wholeheartedly involved, the next 3 people in order of involvement (Numbers 5, 6, and 7 in our ranked list) tended not to be as passionate about the work for its own sake, viewing it more as a duty necessitated by the threat of cancer. Nevertheless, these peo- ple routinely followed their personal program, and over time brought about pronounced psychological change. These 3 differed from one another in their personality and style of work. Number 5 was a reserved person, conscientious, without being excited by the work, although she valued it highly:

> *"I wake up each morning thinking what am I going to do today for myself (relaxing, meditation, etc.) and when shall I do it. I know it is the most important thing to do in my life at the moment."*

She experienced considerable personal change, describing improved self-worth, greater ability to balance her own needs with those of others, more self-expression and awareness, and improved relationships.

> *"I feel I have confronted certain bad habits (such as being a perfectionist, always wanting to have control over my life, and keeping busy all the time) already and am working on many other things."*

She was one of 2 patients in the study (the other being Number 1 on the involvement scale), who, against medical expectations, have had complete remissions of their cancer for some 10 years.

A second member of this cluster was highly anxious, and fear about his disease drove him to dedicated and regular self-help practice (Number 6). By contrast, the third member (Number 7) appeared highly self-confident and calm in face of difficult news and successive surgeries. She chose to avoid overt expression of emotion or psychological self-analysis, but maintained a regular practice of meditation and related techniques, such as relaxation and visualization.

The defining feature of the remaining 2 members in the "highly involved" group (Numbers 8 and 9 on the list) was a tendency to pursue their own agendas. Although dedicated to their self-help practice, they were less open than the other highly involved people to investigating all aspects of their lives. For example, although the homework of Number 9 suggested serious conflicts with her children, she was unwilling to discuss it in any depth with the group. She also considered herself a spiritual person, but was not open to discussions on the topic.

"Some of my contempt for a certain kind of 'spirituality' is not only about its pretentiousness, but also because it seems closed to me."

Moderately Involved People

The next 5 patients in the ranked list were classed as "moderately involved." They were still active in applying self-help strategies but had less ability or willingness to apply themselves. Two of them (Numbers 10 and 13) had difficulty sustaining self-help work beyond an intermittent involvement. Number 10 seesawed between enthusiastic outbursts of activity and periods of depleted relapse. Her most active work was in the spiritual area, where she gained a very strong spiritual feeling and sense of connection. The other member of this cluster (Number 13), felt victimized by her cancer. She believed it "should have not happened to her," and these feelings periodically undermined her resolve to stick with her program:

"Disappointment is the main theme of my life: [my husband] dying, getting cancer, not being cured. I must turn that around."

The remaining 3 "moderately involved" people were all women who had evident blocks to emotional self-expression that seemed to restrict their openness and willingness to change.

"I don't seem to be able to believe that my life is threatened."

"I wouldn't be prepared to take 6 months and do only this self-healing work; the benefits are not sufficiently clear. . . . If there was anything that guaranteed healing, I would probably do that all the time," but I'm *"unwilling to devote 8 hours a day on self-help work."*

All had a tendency to approach things in a very rational way, were not emotionally expressive in the group or in their homework, and tended to withdraw in potentially emotional situations. For example, Number 11 was unable or unwilling to look for any negativity in her thinking. She was reluctant to try drawing, reporting that she "didn't see the need" for fantasy or guided imagery, was ambivalent about asking friends for support, and felt she "shouldn't need" the support of the group.

Minimally Involved People

Eight of the patients were minimally involved in self-help work and were clustered into three further subgroups. "Rejecters" were 2 high-achieving professionals who rejected the need to change, and the notion that the state of their minds could make a difference to their experience, let alone to the physiological regulation of their cancers (both, however, continued to attend and value the emotional support of the group). Three quotes from the writings of Number 20:

> "I'm not going to be a new person . . . I don't have any faith in the process. I am far from unhappy with my current balance of mind and spirit, so why change what works quite well?"

> "I chose not to do this exercise since I see no more point in it for me than previously. . . . . It is just that I believe such problems do not refract upon my illness."

> "Once I go out into the world, I tend to become absorbed by it, to the detriment of homework."

Two further members of the low involvement group, whom we labelled "detached" (Numbers 19 and 22), also seemed skeptical of the power of their minds to make a difference, although they did not actively reject the approach. Their skepticism prevented their getting seriously involved, however. One (Number 19) had pancreatic cancer and died early, although only after several months of fair health. The other (Number 22) represents the only exception to the rule that all in the "low involvement" group died within 2 years of study entry. She had an infant daughter, to whom she wished to devote as much time as possible, although she would do her meditation daily, without apparent enthusiasm.

"I use her [daughter] as my excuse for not doing more self-help [work]."

The remaining 4 individuals appeared to be unable to focus effectively on their healing work because of longstanding patterns of behaviour that were apparent at entry to the study. Two struggled with self-esteem (Numbers 15 and 17); a sense of helplessness and profound feelings of personal unworthiness undermined their efforts. For example,

"I think I am up against a personal trait that I have had for as long as I can remember, which is to study an endeavour sometimes to the point of exhaustion before attempting anything. I'm afraid I may do something wrong, or may fail in my attempt, thereby making myself look foolish or stupid . . . despite all of the encouragement I get from you and the group, I continue in this pattern."

However, in spite of his self doubts, this man still reported "seeing great changes in [my] life with family; everyone is closer, showing concern for one another."

After his death, his wife told us,

"The last weeks and months were wonderful; there was much love between [us]."

Two others (Numbers 16 and 18) expressed high levels of anger and resentment, which appeared to block their openness to change and ability to work. For example,

"I wish my sister and friends would visit me more often. I would like our nanny to stop telling me about all of her problems and make more of an effort to resolve her differences with my husband. The related stress about these things takes away a lot of energy that I could direct toward healing. I wish my husband would recognize and stop hindering offers of help from others and be more sympathetic and compassionate when I'm not feeling well."

WHAT HAS THIS STUDY TAUGHT US?

I hope the excerpts quoted above from patients' writings (homework) have conveyed some idea of the richness of the picture that can be built up when we use this approach to study how people may adapt to a cancer diagnosis when offered psychological help. Imagine 50 to 100 pages of such self-revelation from most subjects, coupled with weekly 2.5-hour meetings over a year, and you will see that we investigators were privileged to get a rather intimate look at the lives of individuals striving to cope with and survive cancer. In comparison, I believe it is fair to say we have learned very little from the 11 published trials, discussed in chapter 4, on the effects of different therapies on survival. I would include our own randomized trial, one of the 11, in that criticism. Such trials will eventually be needed, to confirm that the therapy is a causal factor, but for the present, we need much more exploratory work of this kind. From this small, Healing Journey study, we have learned many of the qualities that may well promote longer survival. Favourable patterns are: having sufficient flexibility and dedication to make an active response to the diagnosis, which entails changes in habits of thought and activity; practising self-control strategies like relaxation, meditation, mental imaging, cognitive monitoring, and becoming involved in a search for meaning in one's life. Obstacles to doing well can be found at a number of points on the model (Figure 5.2). Patients' defensive style may leave little room for change; such inflexibility is commonly associated with low self-esteem or, alternatively, with a fixed world view that the subject sees no reason to alter. There may be skepticism about the potential impact of psychological self-regulation techniques, or about one's ability to apply them. Application to the work is often pre-empted by other activities seen to be more important or more immediately appealing. Positive experiences from applying the techniques may be lacking, diminishing motivation. A need for personal control can be so strong as to lead to the rejection of recommended changes. Meaning may be habitually sought outside the person, rather than through internal searching, and there may be strong contrary views about the validity of spiritual ideas.

Caveats must be noted. This is one small experiment requiring replication. We are currently engaged in another similar, although larger, study for which the final analysis is planned for 2005–2006; current indications are that the life-prolonging effect is still present, although not as strongly as in the experiment just described. It is already clear that there are, once again, several "remarkable survivors." Confirmation is needed from other scientists as well. However, I am confident that the relationship between the mental attitudes we have described and living longer is a real one, not only from this study, but because the findings agree so well with extensive clinical observations by ourselves and other clinicians. My personal experience of cancer and with psychological and spiritual self-help buttress this understanding. The lay reader, perhaps desperate for ways to help herself, should note carefully that we have described a small group of people, some of whom were willing to make healing work the top priority of their lives. Our conclusions cannot be generalized to less-motivated people, and you must be clear that even high dedication to this kind of self-help does not guarantee prolongation of life, let alone "cure"; such desirable outcomes can be seen only as possibilities as yet, and much more work is needed to understand the process of mind-assisted healing and its limitations. However, you can be assured that, with responsible guidance, your quality of life (and dying, it needs to be said), are almost certain to be much enhanced.

In speaking about this work I often encounter quite angry reactions from professionals of various backgrounds. The problem is not usually the data, although some do not accept that we have adequately accounted for medical factors, even with the "blind raters," who predicted survival just as well as the main rating team, but without knowing the patients or their medical histories. Instead the objection is along the lines sketched out in chapter 1: that we should not offer "false hope," encouraging people to try to help themselves, in case they try and "fail," or blame themselves for not trying hard enough. I think there are a number of factors contributing to this criticism. First is likely to be ignorance of the potential that we all have for psychological and spiritual growth, and of the immense personal value of this work, cancer or no cancer. Many in the culture do understand this, but we are still a minority, and it is likely that the only sure way to realize the benefits of, for example, regular meditation, is to do it. Second, as suggested in chapter 1, a lot of people in the mental health professions may, in fact, have an inkling that a degree of healing is possible through the mind, but feel that it is not practical or appealing to try to invoke this potential in clients. Of course the philosophy of self-help must be responsibly presented, without making unsupportable claims. It is true that people in desperate need will often place unwarranted reliance on any method that seems to offer a chance of cure; this problem applies as much to medical treatments as to psychological help. Yet the mental benefits of teaching people to help themselves through their own minds are indisputable, by contrast with the often harsh side effects of medical treatment. I would say to critics, please be open-minded; investigate the field before condemning it; try the mind–body techniques for yourself; be aware that by ridiculing this approach to patients you may fall into the opposite error of "false disempowerment"!

Finally, let us recognize that we have barely begun to investigate the larger issue of the possible impact of mental change on physical disease. In our experiments I have adopted the strategy of working with highly motivated people who will "take the ball and run with it." The aim has been to demonstrate *potential*. Once that is accepted, many more will be interested and motivated to try to help themselves. Obviously, many people in the community will need much more help to achieve a level of self-help comparable to the "highly involved" individuals I have described here. For example, we could envisage a 3-month retreat in a country setting staffed by knowledgeable helpers, life for that time being devoted to healing work. It may sound utopian; it is what I did myself on receiving a diagnosis of cancer, and it would be within the reach of many people, if the value of this kind of dedicated action were understood. The expense is less than that of spending more than a few days in hospital, and most would accept the disruption to their affairs if it brought months or years of extra life.

SUMMARY

I have outlined a stepwise program of psychological therapy, the Healing Journey program, that offers instruction in how to help oneself when faced with cancer (or other serious disease). A research study was conducted with 22 patients in this program, using a design that was different from that of the trials approach reported in the last chapter. We related the efforts that *individuals* made to the duration of their survival. With this method it was possible to demonstrate that those people with serious cancers who became highly involved in self-help lived much longer than medically expected. Two had complete, 8- to 10-year remissions of disease. Other individuals who were not strongly committed to self-help died about as medically predicted. The difference in attitudes between "highly involved" and less involved people was quite striking, and has been illustrated with quotes from the writings of the study subjects. This formal study supports several decades of clinical observations that have come to a similar conclusion: psychological and spiritual growth work seems to prolong life, for at least some people. However, conclusions must be guarded at present: I've discussed some of the limitations of the work, and the reactions it sometimes provokes.

REFERENCEES

1. Cunningham, A. J. (2000). *The healing journey: Overcoming the crisis of cancer.* (2nd ed.). Toronto: Key Porter.
   Cunningham, A. J. (2002). Bringing spirituality into your healing journey. Toronto: Key Porter.
2. Cunningham, A. J., Edmonds, C. V. I., Phillips, C., Soots, K. I., Hedley, D., & Lockwood, G. A. (2000). A prospective, longitudinal study of the relationship of psychological work to duration of survival in patients with metastatic cancer. *Psycho-oncology, 9,* 323–339.
   Cunningham, A. J., Phillips, C., Lockwood, G. A., Hedley, D., & Edmonds, C. V. I. (2000). Association of involvement in psychological self help with longer survival in patients with metastatic cancer: An exploratory study. *Advances in Mind–Body Medicine, 16,* 276–294.
   Cunningham, A. J., Phillips, C., Stephen, J., & Edmonds, C. (2002). Fighting for life: A qualitative analysis of the process of psychotherapy-assisted self-help in patients with metastatic cancer. *Integrative Cancer Therapies, 1*(2), 146–161.
3. Details of our experiment can be found on our website www.healingjourney.ca, and the papers can be located by clicking on the "Research" link.
4. A more detailed account, with information about the medical conditions of the participants, is given in Cunningham, Phillips, Stephen, & Edmonds (2002).

Chapter 6

The Qualities of Long Survivors

The 22 subjects in the last chapter afforded us a privileged insight into their fight for life against disease diagnosed as terminal. We were able, in the study, to meet with most of them every week for a year, and to read and hear intimate descriptions of their feelings, reflections on their condition, and accounts of self-help efforts. Those clinicians who undertake long-term psychological therapy with people who have metastatic cancers may gain similar insights, but there are features of a rigorous study like this that enable us to go beyond the usual clinical impressions and derive conclusions with some confidence. While we are currently undertaking another study of this kind, it is my hope that other researchers will also see the advantages of following individuals in such an intensive way, and will provide their own descriptions of any relationship they uncover between psychological adaptive styles and survival. What is the next step? We might ask, "What would be an ideal experiment designed to document the kinds of psychological change, and the eventual state of mind achieved, that assist people with life-threatening cancers (or other disease) to live substantially longer?"

An ideal study might begin by recruiting a large number (hundreds) of patients just diagnosed with incurable cancers. Careful medical histories would be compiled for each individual at the time of entry to the study, and predictions as to likely survival time made by experts for each participant. Psychological therapy would be provided, and a dynamic psychological "profile" obtained for everyone, by collecting data from interviews or therapy sessions (chapter 5) over a period of years. Those who greatly outlived their predicted lifespan would be of special interest, of course. The data from the interviews with these people after they had achieved this "exceptional" status would yield insights into the kinds of change that accompanied prolonged survival, and could be contrasted with the profiles of others who had not been so fortunate. Given a framework like this, it would be possible to determine whether, or in what respects, long-surviving patients were unusual or unique, and while it would not prove that the psychology caused the long survival, there would be a strong indication that it did in fact make a difference. Such an experiment is obviously extremely costly, perhaps impossible to do completely, but it is feasible to attempt parts of it. The study reported in the last chapter was one part, albeit on a small scale: it involved describing the psychological adjustments made by a relatively small number of patients over a year, and as we saw, there appeared to be a relationship between the nature of the adjustments and survival duration. The study I want to report in this chapter explores another piece of the ideal—interviews with individuals many years after they have outlived their prognoses. This time, instead of following the process of striving to heal, we are viewing their healing through a different window, by taking a snapshot of the state they eventually achieve. The subjects we have recruited for this purpose are all graduates from our Healing Journey therapy program, and most were in the study of chapter 5 or are participants in its current replication, so it is possible to contrast them with their peers who have not outlived expectancies.

To understand how this is an advance over the interview studies on remarkable survivors described in chapter 3, let us review some of the limitations of those earlier, more anecdotal reports, weaknesses that are important because they have caused the work to be dismissed by most professionals in the field.

1. The most serious difficulty, often cited by critics, is that if we interview only "remarkable survivors" plucked, as it were, out

of a much larger population of unknown size, we can't tell if they are in any way unusual psychologically. We need some comparison with the profiles of others who fail to survive. If we can determine that long survivors have unusual or unique psychological attributes from the start, it becomes much more probable that these attributes contributed to their fortunate outcomes, whereas if many other people share these qualities, this is much less likely to be the case. We encountered a similar problem in chapter 1 when briefly discussing claims for magical dietary or other "alternative" remedies: if someone ingests substance X and recovers unexpectedly, he or she is likely to attribute the cure to that substance; but if we learn that 100 other people took the same remedy and failed to survive, we see that the first person's happy outcome was probably not caused by X.

2. There was, in most cases, no thorough documentation of the medical histories of the interviewees. When the subjects for interview are obtained by advertising for them, there is a risk of attracting a tiny minority of people who are medically unusual, perhaps with mistaken diagnoses or anomalous disease; hence the need for thorough checks. Although such people are probably rare, there may well be a few of them among the thousands of people who have at some time been diagnosed with metastatic cancer in any large metropolitan centre. Some of these people may have survived a long time because they did not, in fact, have a serious cancer, in which case it would be misleading to link their psychological adaptation with their good outcome.

3. In the early studies, subjects were not known to the investigators apart from a single interview, or at most a small number of interviews, conducted long after their diagnosis and recovery. It is difficult to be sure, under these circumstances, that what people report accurately represents their thoughts and actions during previous years.

These design weaknesses do not disprove the idea that the mental state found in these patients was related to their long survival, but do make that inference much less compelling. However, the common factors found among such long-surviving individuals suggest some kind of true relationship, as I discussed in chapter 3. Could we do a more reliable experiment of this kind, and compare the results with those of the earlier, more impressionistic accounts?

I'm going to describe the results of current, ongoing research in which we interviewed and analyzed the statements of 10 long-surviving graduates of the Healing Journey program (and I acknowledge here the skilled help of Kim Watson, psychological associate). A technical report on this study has recently been published,[1] with details on the nature of their cancers, and duration of survival beyond that predicted by the panel, as well as a qualitative analysis of what they said in their interviews. We also interviewed two comparison groups. The first of these included 6 subjects who had metastatic disease, and had applied to enter the program, but had not yet begun in it, or had done similar work elsewhere. We expected that these people would reflect a state of mind more usual in the population, which we were interested to compare with that of our 10 exceptional program graduates. The second comparison group comprised the 6 individuals who were at the bottom end of our "observed/expected" hierarchy from the experiment of the last chapter; that is, they were the 6 individuals who showed the lowest survival, in comparison with that medically predicted, out of the 22 studied. Since all died many years ago, we examined their home assignment writings and therapist notes from the period when they attended the weekly group therapy sessions. We expected that the psychological profiles of these individuals would also contrast with those of the long survivors.

In brief, the 10 people with extended survival have, at the time of writing, lived from 4 to about 14 years longer than predicted by a panel of experts. They have had a range of medically incurable, usually metastatic diagnoses: breast cancer (5 cases), and one each of colorectal, malignant melanoma, multiple myeloma, lymphoma, and uterine cancers. The picture we will derive from this investigation applies most directly to groups of people like the cancer patients we interviewed: all were middle-class people, all Caucasian, and all in the age range of 48 to 70 years of age. Nine were women. We can't necessarily assume that other groups of survivors would show similar characteristics, although as we will see, there was good agreement between what was found with these people and the various anecdotal reports in the literature.

While this is by no means an ideal investigation, many of the earlier design problems have been solved: in particular, these people were all survivors from the Healing Journey program and well known to us, in most cases over many years, before the interviews were done. Thus we can be confident that what they said reflected their enduring attitudes. Six were participants in the study described in chapter 5, or in its current replication. Thus we can also be confident, from the chart reviews by a panel of experts, that they were not medically anomalous at the time when we enrolled them—they were not identified as "unusual" or "exceptional" until several years later, by which time they had substantially outlived their predicted life expectancies.

Perhaps most important, we can document that the long-surviving interviewees in the present study were psychologically unlike most of their non-surviving peers during the first year of their struggles with cancer, being much more involved in their self-help than those who failed to survive. This strengthens the likelihood that their long survival was somehow related to their psychology, an argument for which there was no independent evidence in the early studies. Nevertheless, they were not unique psychologically: some other equally involved people did not outlive their prognosis to the same extent, although such individuals were not numerous. The fact that we do not find an invariable association between high involvement and prolonged survival is hardly surprising; other factors must also play a role, perhaps psychological attributes that we do not yet recognize, and also, most certainly, the biology of the disease. As noted earlier, the medical/biological aspects of a cancer may be so strong in many cases as to rapidly overwhelm the patient, regardless of psychological adjustment.

Because our long survivors were part of a larger study group, we are also able to test whether people with relatively low involvement ever outlive their predicted lifespan. The case for an association between involvement and survival would be stronger if they do not. In the study reported in the last chapter we found that patients with involvement scores in the lowest third do not live much longer than medically predicted, only 1 having outlived the prediction by as much as 2 years. Exceptional survival thus seems not to be an entirely chance event, but to correlate strongly with certain psychological attributes.

Thus from our data so far, we can say that patients who survive in "remarkable" fashion are not average psychologically; they tend to have demonstrated high involvement early in (and throughout) their struggle with cancer. Although such involvement does not guarantee long survival, highly involved people seem to live longer than average, and low involvement is almost always associated with relatively short survival. In all previous investigations of this kind, there was no possibility of relating long survival to unusual psychological characteristics in this way. Now, as we move to the next stage of the work, describing the qualities of people at a point where they have outlived life expectancies by many years, we can be more confident that some real association exists between their psychological profiles and their long survival. In all probability, their engagement with their own healing has contributed to the mental state they have ultimately reached. We will see that there are many common features among these people, and that they do in fact resemble closely the remarkable survivors described in chapter 3, lending credibility to the growing picture of mental states contributing to favourable medical outcome. Later in the chapter we will put these observations together with a theory by L. Temoshok, to generate a simple but evidence-based account of the psychological factors that may contribute to disease and healing.

WHAT THE LONG SURVIVORS TOLD US

In the interviews, which were 60 to 90 minutes long, we wanted people to tell us what was important to them, without imposing our own ideas. So my first question was simply, "What are your thoughts and feelings as you review your cancer experience, and how has it affected your life?" after which the interviewee spoke for as long as he or she liked. I would ask for clarification and elaboration of specific points, but was basically guided by the person I was interviewing. The conversations were taped, and a summary transcription made. A technical paper based on this study is in preparation; I offer a summary here.

A dominant theme emerging from a comparison of transcripts was that these people felt they were now living as they wanted to live, in contrast to a more obligation-driven existence before cancer. All 10 asserted that they were doing what they valued in life, and making their own choices. Examples of this autonomy:

"My life is different now, and many of the differences are quite positive ones for me, resting more, doing the things I love, spending time with people I love. Those are things I had difficulty making time for before."

"I certainly gave up things that I was doing because I felt I ought to, and I think that it propelled me to a new level of self-examination and self-awareness."

"I don't see it as a gift, but it certainly was cancer that made me step back and reflect on what I want to do, and why I want to do it, and to make better choices for myself and enjoy life a little bit more."

"I really feel I used to put a lot of demands on myself. I used to worry about being perfect in everything that I did. I'm still somewhat of a person that wants to please, and I'm being very selective in terms of what I'm doing right now."

In 5 of the 10, the point was made that life had been simplified to allow this pursuit of the desired way of being:

"I've decided not to go back to work. I've never really given myself the opportunity to heal in the sense that I'm noncommittal to anybody, that I can just devote the time to myself. In doing that, my direction has changed."

By contrast, these themes were much more weakly expressed in the comparison groups of people interviewed before starting the therapy, or among those from the Healing Journey experiment (chapter 5) whose survival was not prolonged. More characteristic among these individuals was a sense of confusion, or lack of direction:

"I have a hard time even identifying what I need and then putting it into place."

"The constant certainty has been being frightened, being terrified, feeling helpless and hopeless."

The self-help techniques that had been learned in the Healing Journey program were highly valued and were used by all the long survivors, although they tended to be employed "as needed," that is, as stressful circumstances arose, rather than daily:

"I've realized that what works for us today is a changing thing; sometimes meditation is where I need to be, sometimes it's journalling, sometimes it's just quiet reflection, sometimes walking meditation. I've learned to look and say, 'Is this what I need right now?'"

"Visualization and meditation helped me at that time, and I still do it, not faithfully every day, but it's a great help a couple of times a week, or anytime you feel stressed you can meditate and try to still your mind."

Meditation was singled out as a technique of particular value:

"Now when I can quiet my mind and I meditate and I'm still, what comes through is more direction, peacefulness, a feeling of

*love. That inner space is very valuable to me. I think that's where
I connect with what's beyond myself."*

Eight of the survivors volunteered that cancer itself was now much less important in their lives, and although all but 3 of them still had some evidence of active disease, medical advice was viewed as only one facet of their continuing health maintenance. They had learned to take responsibility for their health themselves, and tended to see the cancer diagnosis as more of a motivator than a threat:

"One thing that I have learned is how important it is to have a sense of control about my treatment process. I need to know what's going on, and I need to know that what I do can affect that and that I have part in the decision-making process."

"I seem to be telling myself it doesn't matter what the doctors say, you've got your own journey. You can't rely on them to tell you what you're going to do when you really do know what you're going to do in your own mind."

The experience of overcoming a serious cancer, for at least some years, left all of these individuals with a sense that their lives had changed profoundly for the better. Among the improvements described were increased peacefulness, joy, more self-understanding, and an ability to take obstacles in their stride:

"I've experienced a peacefulness and a joy that I'm not having to run after the whole world and catch it by the tail. I don't have to do anymore, I just have to learn to be."

"It [cancer] truly, truly was one of the richest things that ever happened to me. If I hadn't gotten cancer I would still be racing through life doing everything perfectly, and everything so well organized, and life is so much richer and meaningful."

Relations with other people were much improved, tolerance and loving acceptance being frequently mentioned, a lessening of their need to control others, more ready expression of feelings, and often a specific motivation to help others:

"There are patterns that I see in myself now that I didn't see before, and I think I'm able slowly, slowly to notice the patterns that I get stuck in more quickly when they happen, especially in relationships with other people. Right now I'm at a point where I frequently notice it, and I sometimes can respond differently or create space in there to let myself react without jumping in a habitual way that I always did."

"Since the cancer I've been able to talk about things as opposed to holding them in. I guess maybe I used to feel that what I had to say wasn't that important, and now maybe it is."

Finally, a greater sense of meaning in life and connection to a larger order or spiritual dimension was noted by almost all the long survivors. Gratitude, as much for the greatly improved quality of life as for the long survival, was expressed in almost all cases:

"When I started on my journey, I knew God was there, but I hadn't connected in the sense that I could communicate with him. I wasn't aware of what was going on around me. Now a lot more things come naturally to me, in the sense of giving and being able to sit alone and connect with God, being able to talk to him, being able to see messages that are sent to me."

"I've been given so much from friends and people, the doctors I've had, that this coping skills course was here in Toronto: it could have been in Alaska and I wouldn't have had access to it. I couldn't have gotten the groundwork then that I need. I'm grateful just about every day."

At this point I have to admit to an initial feeling of disappointment with the results of these interviews. Being someone who sees the spiritual search, and personal growth generally, as the major purpose of life, I hoped, even expected, that this would be the dominant theme in our subjects. What we did find was less elevated: people living the way they wanted to live. However, in no instance did this mean a life of mindless pleasure-seeking! There was evidence of a greater meaning in life, or self-transcendence in the form of stronger relationship to something beyond the self, which for some took the form of spiritual connection, and for others was more aesthetic or interpersonal. Using their enhanced knowledge of inner psychological processes, these people were able to maintain a pattern to their days that brought peace and satisfaction. On reflection, I see that this result, which at first appeared a bit pedestrian, is actually hopeful, because if it is true that the approach to life that our subjects displayed is life-sparing, then it is within the reach of almost any motivated person. It is also, incidentally, the pattern described as healing by the very perceptive and experienced clinical psychologist Lawrence LeShan in his book *Cancer as a Turning Point* (referred to in chapter 1).

INTEGRATION OF STUDIES ON LONG SURVIVORS

I've already alluded to the close similarity in results between the interviews of long survivors from our program and the various interview studies describing people who claim prolonged survival (chapter 3). The reader may wish to refer back to Figure 3.1. Increased "autonomy," meaning perceiving the freedom to make one's own choices in life, predominated in both sets of analyses. The enhanced experience of joy, self-understanding, appreciation of life and sense of its value were also common to both. The "remarkable survivor" studies often reported that their participants had greater self-acceptance and esteem; this achievement is difficult to deduce from a single interview, but is an attribute we can confirm from our acquaintance with our interviewees over a prolonged time. Greater tolerance, and love for others, and freer expression of feelings—attributes that are closely tied to self–esteem—were found both by us and in the earlier reports. Substantial change, assisted by a variety of self-help techniques, was almost always noted, although the "spiritual-existential" shift remarked on in a number of the earlier descriptions of remarkable survivors, while present, was less dramatic in our interviews. It may be that when people fighting for their lives can access a structured program, the healing change becomes more gradual and reliable, whereas in people not given such help, a more sudden and perhaps less common kind of sudden shift in attitudes is needed to generate the same impact on the physiology. Overall, it seems fair to say that the central change in the people described in all of these studies is towards greater authenticity in their lives.

We can add to this growing picture of survivorship the information from the prospective study reported in chapter 5. There the perspective was slightly different: we were following people with presumed fatal disease at a relatively early stage of their struggle. Because of the opportunity for intensive observation of these patients over a prolonged period, we were able to directly observe the qualities they brought with them at the start: their openness to change, expectancy that healing was possible, determination to help themselves—attitudes about which we are less certain when they are simply reported years after the fact, as in retrospective interviews. The focus in the Healing Journey study was then on what people actually thought and did over the year of observation, and we documented the degree to which they were motivated to apply the psychological and spiritual methods taught. Already at the end of the year, however, many of the same benefits were seen as in the later interviews of those who subsequently survived a long time, such as increased joy, peace, acceptance of others, and discovery of increased meaningfulness of life.

Figure 6.1 is an integration of the results from reports on "remarkable survivors" (chapter 3), from the Healing Journey study of chapter 5, and from the interviews of long survivors described in this chapter. Those who enjoy prolonged survival exhibit an initial openness and determination that drives them to help themselves. The Healing Journey study charted the dedicated efforts that resulted. As a result of these efforts, a more "authentic" self emerged, already evident after 1 year of healing work, and more fully documented in the interviews of survivors some years later, or of people from the wider community who claimed to have greatly outlived their prognoses. The changed individual now feels entitled to choose how to live, displays much greater acceptance of others (without allowing herself

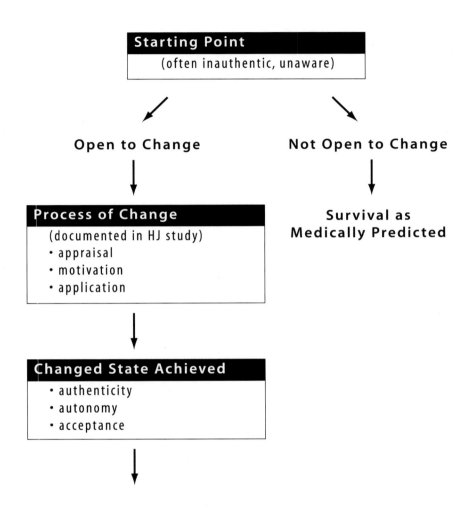

FIGURE 6.1 *The process of change in long survivors: an integration of the results from reports on "remarkable survivors," from the Healing Journey study of chapter 5, and from the interviews of long survivors described in this chapter.*

to be imposed upon), and enjoys a more peaceful and meaningful life. These qualities reinforce one another, of course: learning to accept others aids self-acceptance, which enhances the sense of autonomy. Learning to make one's own choices increases the experience of the authenticity of one's life.

What would a critic say to all this? That these studies are small, have a subjective component (the interviewer often needs to interpret what the subject says), and are restricted in their generalizability to a rather unusual sub-population of people with cancer. How would I respond? That convergence of evidence from several studies is always compelling in science. That the Healing Journey studies and the "interview study" reported above, although small, do not suffer from serious technical weaknesses, as a detailed reading of our peer-reviewed, published papers will show. We acknowledge that it is not possible to be sure that the psychological changes *caused* the longer survival, although no convincing alternatives have been offered by critics. The generalizability of all of these studies is certainly low, meaning that conclusions apply most directly to people similar to those who presented themselves, and results may or may not be reproducible in different populations. Studies of long survivors and the process of healing change need to be done in many settings, with differing groups of patients; when so little is known in a field, this kind of discovery-oriented or theory-building approach is much more appropriate than the theory-testing imperative that drives much current medical research (see chapter 4). No doubt, modifications and extensions of the current description will unfold. I will be very surprised if the overall conclusion is wrong, however, because it makes such good, developmental *sense*, a point to which we now turn.

A DEVELOPMENTAL LOOK AT CANCER AND HEALING

There is one more, important set of evidence to add to our growing, integrative picture. Recall the work of Lydia Temoshok (chapter 4), who defined a Type C adaptive style, an attitude of "niceness" and denial of one's own needs, common among people with cancer, and associated with faster progression of the disease. We can add to this the reasonably consistent evidence for a link between repression of emotion and higher risk of cancer progression. Temoshok's view of the role of mind in development of cancer is that the early development of this self-protective, placatory style of relating to the world puts a great strain on the regulator systems of the body, such as the immune system. This demand makes the body less able to resist or control later onset of disease. She also suggests that the logical way to use the mind to fight cancer is to try to reverse the harmful elements of this self-denying style. That is also the conclusion Lawrence LeShan draws from his clinical experience, as we have seen. Now, note how this is precisely what the long survivors have done, in the studies just described. They have become determined to live life as they wished to, as opposed to always trying to please others. Through their work and change they have understood the load they were imposing on themselves, seen its irrationality, and worked hard to reverse it. As a result, far from becoming selfish monsters, they achieved an acceptance of self and others, a joyful appreciation of life, and a sense of meaning and fulfilment in life that most "well" people would envy.

This is what I mean by the model or hypothesis "making sense." There is a mirrored symmetry between the concepts of what promotes cancer and the evidence on what prolongs survival (Figure 6.2 puts together diagrammatically the development and the reversing of mental states that promote cancer). Furthermore, the model does not depend on the correctness of the specific details of mental states that are proposed as promoting development or later retardation of cancer growth. The predisposing psychological factors might not always be Type C. The important point is that some early distortion of the healthy, authentic adaptation to life occurs, and that this causes strain. The neurophysiologist Bruce McEwen calls this "allostatic load."[2] If we grow up unduly fearful, or for that matter with any other kind of maladaptation, like constant anger or depression, we may place a lifelong stress on the regulators of our health, in particular the cardiovascular, immune, respiratory, nervous, and detoxifica-

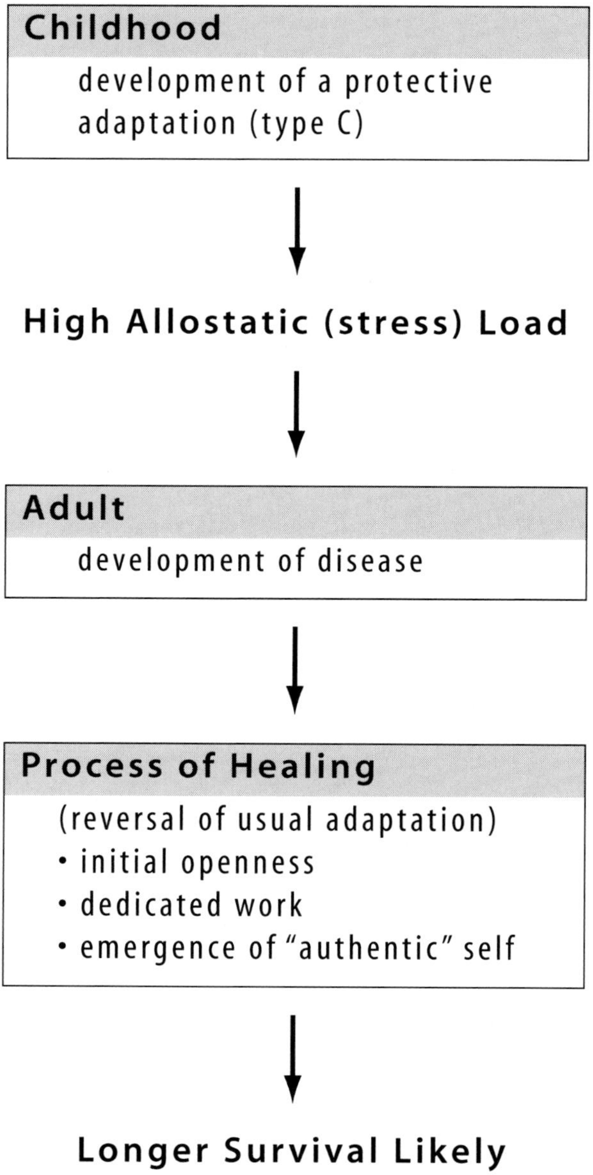

Childhood

development of a protective
adaptation (type C)

High Allostatic (stress) Load

Adult

development of disease

Process of Healing

(reversal of usual adaptation)
• initial openness
• dedicated work
• emergence of "authentic" self

Longer Survival Likely

FIGURE 6.2 *A simple developmental chart of possible mental contributions to the onset and healing of cancer*

tion systems of the body, and on the cellular-level micro-regulators that they influence in turn (chapter 2). Note that this is a general theory, applicable to many diseases, not just to cancer. For example, the theory would predict that the Type A personality develops early and places strain particularly on the cardiovascular system. It would further predict that diminishing the heightened risk of heart disease (although probably not established damage) could be accomplished by reversing the distorted adaptation—learning to react to challenges with tolerance instead of anger. There is some evidence for the success of this approach, not yet universally accepted (chapter 2). This explanation of events is simple and makes sense. It does not claim, simplistically, that "the mind *cures* cancer" or any other disease: the prediction merely is that to the extent that the mind and its distortions are important, reversal of the harmful adaptation will be helpful. The extent of the contribution of mind has to be established by experiment, and one way to do this is to evaluate the effects of psychological change, assisted by therapy.

There should be nothing in this model to offend even the most materialistic of readers, or to generate any feelings of blame or guilt among people with cancer. I am not invoking any esoteric "powers of mind," simply suggesting that bodily health is promoted by optimizing the health of the mind, a return to an equilibrium that has been disrupted early in life for reasons outside one's individual control. This trait is more marked in some people than in others; those individuals carrying the greatest allostatic (stress) load may be more likely to contract a variety of diseases in adult life. Many factors (such as genetic, environmental, and infectious) contribute to disease, and consequently, many modes of treatment may be helpful; working through the mind to reduce strain is one important mode.

SUMMARY

While chapter 5 focused on the thoughts and actions of individuals as they were fighting for their lives against metastatic cancer, this chapter examines the influence of mental states on prolongation of life in a different way, through interviews with patients some years after they have outlived their medically predicted lifespan. I report on our own interview study of survivors who have taken the Healing Journey program, then show the strong similarities that exist between what these individuals report and the various accounts from "remarkable survivors" discussed in chapter 3. We then put this information together with Temoshok's theory, that cancer is more likely to occur in those people who developed, in childhood, a particular kind of placatory and emotionally repressed coping style. We see that what the long survivors appear to have done is to reverse this way of adapting to the world, claiming instead their right to make their own decisions about how to live their lives. This enhanced authenticity is associated with greater acceptance of others, and of oneself, and leads to a more peaceful and meaningful experience of life. It also appears to help people live longer, as well as better.

REFERENCES

1. Cunningham, A.J., & Watson, K. (2004). How psychological therapy may prolong survival in cancer patients: New evidence and a simple theory. *Integrative Cancer Therapies, 3*, 214–229.
2. McEwen, B. S. (1998). Protective and damaging effects of stress mediators: Allostasis and allostatic load. *New England Journal of Medicine, 338*, 171–179.
   McEwen, B. S., & Lasley, E. N. (2002). *The end of stress as we know it.* Washington, DC: Joseph Henry.

Chapter 7

A Summary, and Future Directions

The discussion to this point about a possible impact of mind on healing from cancer has been based on what we know or can reasonably infer from available evidence. In this last section I want to be more speculative. We will look first at how spiritual influences may fit into the simple model of mind–cancer discussed in the last chapter, since many people, both throughout history and at present, have viewed this dimension as very important in healing. My earlier book *Bringing Spirituality into Your Healing Journey*[1] is a detailed account of this kind of healing, including many practical exercises. Then we will summarize what we have learned in 2 decades of this healing work, and offer suggestions for further investigation, both by people seeking to help themselves and by those wanting to help others.

THE SPIRITUAL DIMENSION IN HEALING

The spiritual search is an attempt to gain direct experience of our place in, and our relationship to, a transcendent, non-material order, dimension, matrix, intelligence, or power. This order has been given a great variety of names, at different times and in different cultures: the Universal Mind, the Divine, Brahman, the One, the Tao, the Eternal, Yahwe, God. To "transcend" means, literally, to rise above or extend beyond, and the implication here is that the non-material spiritual reality not only goes far beyond what we can perceive with our ordinary senses but also profoundly affects our everyday life. Spirituality is distinguishable from religion, the latter referring to institutionalized systems of ritual, faith, and worship, which are not necessarily concerned with the attempt to gain direct experience of the transcendent.

Spiritual or mystical experience has manifested in similar forms in many cultures in all parts of the world, giving rise to a description of "the perennial philosophy" (a term coined by Spinoza), for which Happold, in his book *Mysticism*,[2] lists the following common features (paraphrased here):

- The world of matter and individual consciousness is only a partial reality and is the manifestation of a Divine Ground or God in which all partial realities have their being.
- Man (humankind) can know this Divine Ground by direct intuition, which is superior to discursive reasoning.
- Although we are chiefly conscious of the separate ego, we can identify with the spark of our divinity within, that is, with that eternal aspect of ourselves, which is part of the Divine Ground.
- It is the chief end of our earthly existence to discover this eternal self.

Traditionally, it has been claimed that being connected to the spiritual realm, to one's "eternal self," promotes healing—of body as well as mind. The problem for those attempting to study healing in a scientific/rational way, the approach we are adopting in this book, is that we currently do not understand how a non-material level or entity could influence events on the material plane. Perhaps the awareness of one's spiritual nature is simply so comforting that it brings about a mental state ideal for healing. Or perhaps there are interactions between the spiritual and the material that use pathways ("subtle energies" is one popular expression) that we don't yet know how to measure. More radically, consciousness may be the "primary" reality, as maintained in some Eastern philosophies, and matter a projection of this consciousness (Table 7.1). In the absence of an agreed conceptual framework, is there something scientists can do at present to investigate the possible importance of spirituality in healing? The most obvious course would seem to be to look for evidence that self-reported spiritual experience is health-promoting—in other words, to treat this as we might any other psychological attribute. There is growing interest in this approach, although most published research to date has used religious observance behaviours (like attendance at church) as a surrogate for spirituality.[3] In the experiments we have been considering in chapters 4 to 6, spirituality was indeed regarded as important by most of the long survivors, and by the most highly involved people in our Healing Journey study. However, it is not possible to disentangle it, in these or other studies so far, from other psychological properties, that is, we cannot be sure that becoming involved in the spiritual search was an essential element, over and above psychological change, in the healing of these people.

Another way to assess the plausibility of the idea that spirituality aids healing is to ask if it fits with our data and evolving theory (shown in Figure 6.2) that the mind promotes healing by reversing earlier psychological habits. The spiritual search, so the mystics tell us, is an attempt to reverse our estrangement from the very ground of our being, which occurs as we grow up into little independent entities, preoccupied with our separate needs. This separation represents the loss of awareness of our true identity. Healing has always been seen, in spiritual traditions, as a process of finding out who we are, rediscovering this identity. This sounds very similar to what our long-surviving patients have been telling us: their central motif was an uncovering of the true self, living according to what was felt most fulfilling, rather than according to old, unexamined habits and dictates. It is also exactly what the spiritual search involves: finding out who we are, and living according to that awareness, only in this case the revelation strikes even deeper; we find that we are not simply material beings but have an essential non-material, or spiritual, nature. In other words, it is the ultimate re-establishing of authenticity! It seems to be the same kind of process that occurs psychologically,

TABLE 7.1   *Range of Views on Possible Healing through Mind*

View of Mind	How Mind Is Related to Body and Illness	View of Cancer, and Potential Healing Impact of Mind
1. Mind is separate, unimportant.	All is given, "out there." Mind is simply a by-product of brain.	Cancer is caused by chance or external agencies. Only external, physical manipulations can affect it. Mind has no effect.
2. Mind creates experience.	The mind observes and interprets, controls behaviour, but affects physiology only in small ways.	As above. Mental change can improve our coping experience, however.
3. Mind is informational correlate of matter	Mind and body are intimately related, not separate; thus events in mind affect physiology.	Mental change makes conditions more or less favourable for cancer development.
4. Mind creates reality.	Mind, which is part of an infinite order (the Divine), creates the world by projection, including body, illness.	Mind can create a different world (apparent "physical" laws, e.g., time and space, are not absolute). Thus it may cure illness.

as people learn and grow, but transferred to the spiritual dimension. Our theory about healing as recovery of authenticity, based on psychological data, thus connects nicely with a philosophy that extends back over millennia. In Figure 7.1 I have added the spiritual dimension to a simplified version of the earlier flow chart to show this symmetry.

WHAT ABOUT ESOTERIC POWERS OF MIND AND SPIRIT?

Are there potentials for healing through the mind that lie outside what we currently understand about mind–body operations. Of course there are: Western psychology, physics, and biology provide only one very limited view of what is possible in the world. Any example of mind affecting matter is potentially relevant to healing; for example, there are many excellent controlled experiments to show that mental intention can affect the output of a computer generating supposedly random numbers (well described in *Margins of Reality* by R. Jahn and B. Dunne).[4] Likewise, instances of mind apparently *dissociating* from matter (excluding pathological dissociation) may have implications for healing. In my clinical practice I quite frequently hear accounts of people having the experience of "leaving their bodies," often while meditating, or around the time of surgery. Analogous "near death experiences" have been documented by many authors. Other paranormal events, like telepathy, precognition, and remote vision—essentially seeing through the eyes of someone at a distance—are also well documented, and point to possibilities for healing by non-Newtonian means, even if skeptics scoff at them. As I described in chapter 2, there are now several good, scientifically acceptable experiments showing a degree of healing in people who are prayed for, without their knowledge (there are also some studies with negative results). Larry Dossey is the physician who has perhaps done most to champion what he calls non-local healing, in a series of books and in his excellent editorials for the new scientific journal *Alternative Therapies.*[5]

Our ideas on what the mind can do to heal the body reflect the prevailing ideology, which in turn is based on metaphysical views (on the nature of reality). Table 7.1 sets out a range of such views. That most commonly held at present is number 1, sometimes called "naive physicalism" or materialism. I have subscribed to number 3 in this book. View number 4 is the mystical position, that our material reality is some kind of projection from our consciousness or mind. It is fascinating, but although esoteric modes of healing may become important to us eventually, as they are already in some cultures (such as through shamanic healing), they are of little practical use unless we can invoke them reliably. Since this approach is not yet acceptable to most Western health care providers, it makes more sense (at least to me) to focus on what we can bring about in a dependable way. The modest degree of healing through making changes in one's mental state that I've described in this book is achievable by most people. It is true that few avail themselves of it as yet, but the pathway towards doing so is reasonably clear, and will become clearer with further research. However, it is unfortunately also the case that personal experience is needed to gain an appreciation of the great power that psychological and spiritual methods have to change our lives. This limitation can set up an initial barrier: one needs the experience of benefit to commit to the self-help work, yet without commitment, it is hard to discover its value.

As I suggested in my earlier book on spirituality and healing, our ability to use our various dimensions in the service of healing depends directly on our awareness and connection with these levels of our being. To use our minds therapeutically, we must be aware of our thoughts and have at least some sense of how they affect our physiology. To invoke spiritual healing, we must be connected spiritually. There is no call to adopt beliefs uncritically—the point is to seek our own understanding and experience, after which we can use it to help ourselves. We must also accept the fact, of course, that there are practical limits to what we can achieve with our minds—the body is a type of machine that will eventually degenerate and die, no matter what we do.

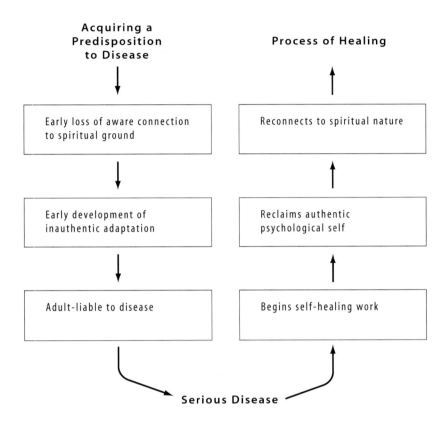

FIGURE 7.1 *The symmetry between possible promoting and healing influences of the mind on cancer. Spiritual disconnection, almost universal among humans, and reconnection as spiritual growth proceeds, can be placed at either end of this pathway.*

POSSIBLE DIRECTIONS FOR FURTHER RESEARCH

While few would deny that the mind has some effect on the body, there is certainly debate about the *extent* of the effect that any healing of the mind can have on the body. Medicine as an organization still tends to downplay, even totally ignore, the possibility that the patient's state of mind is important, although many individual physicians would endorse the idea. Other emerging disciplines, like health psychology or "mind–body medicine," are much more open to it. Some "alternative" practitioners bring the whole idea of mind–body healing into disrepute by making exaggerated claims, unsupported by evidence. In the end it is, or should be, an empirical question, to be settled by investigation, not prejudice. In this next section I want to suggest what might be done next. Here I am addressing primarily the reader who is a health care provider or researcher.

The Key Requirement: Refining Our Understanding of Mental States That Encourage Healing

We need to know much more about the kinds of mental states, and the changes leading up to them, that oppose progression of disease, in cancer and in other chronic conditions. We have barely begun to investigate this matter; discussions on health psychology tend to centre on healthy behaviours, which are only the most obvious expressions of mind–body influences on health (and recall the discussion in chapter 1 about "external" and "internal" pathways). Yet there is a wealth of knowledge, both in the mental health field and in spiritual traditions, about what constitutes a healthy way of being in the world, in other words healthy thinking. We need to connect this with physical well-being, in my opinion.

Since we know very little as yet, we need to put much more of our effort into exploratory approaches. This means remaining open-minded about what is important in people's response to disease, and documenting it by listening closely to them over extended periods, then relating what they say to physical outcomes. Multiple studies of this kind will be needed to build up a reliable picture of healthy mind–body relationships. Anecdotal approaches are not sufficient: we need some variant of the approach outlined in chapters 5 and 6: regular contact and note-taking, followed by qualitative analysis of the verbal data, and by rating these data (putting numbers to them) where we wish to draw quantitative conclusions. Research methods that rely solely on comparing average differences between treatment and control groups are likely to continue to give mixed or null results, because, as I pointed out in chapter 4, people's response to psychological therapy is so variable. However, once we have a better understanding of what helps whom, and how, it will be possible to use statistical methods to control for this variability, and the standard methods used in clinical trials of drugs will then be appropriate to confirm (or deny) a causal role of the therapy.

Our focus at present will thus be more on what people do with any therapeutic help they receive, and much less on the nature of the therapy itself. As we learn more, we will gradually refine our ideas about the undoubtedly complex combinations of mental qualities that matter. Hand in hand with this learning will go the development of methods or plans of assessment that document the extent to which different people make healing changes. Eventually, we should be able to perform a "mind scan" analogous to the current CT scan, that is, to diagnose the extent to which the mental state of people with a chronic disease is helping or hindering them, and recommend appropriate changes! I foresee a time when such monitoring of people's progress towards optimizing the mental aspects of their healing will become routine, just as it is now with physical measurements such as white blood cell counts or liver function tests.

Outcome Measures

To assess the impact of psychological change on disease, one may use a variety of markers, depending on the specific condition: for cancer, blood tests are sometimes available to track tumour growth, or X-ray imagery to determine the size of tumours. These surrogate measures do bring their own uncertainties; we chose lifespan as the most unambiguous index of effect. I would reiterate here, though, that length of life is not necessarily the most important outcome of providing psychological help; the quality of people's lives, their emotional state, their relationships with other people, may matter more in the end. However, if it becomes widely believed that life can be prolonged by the kinds of mental work discussed here, it may have a more persuasive influence on many people—physicians, insurance companies, family members—and the patients themselves, when they are considering whether or not to undertake a program of self-help.

One of the more challenging aspects of research on the ability of mind to affect progression of disease is that it must be longitudinal, that is, we must follow and document what people do over relatively long periods of time, years rather than months (dramatic, sudden healings are so rare as to be almost inaccessible to study). I've put forward the relatively conservative view that the mind has the potential to affect growth of some cancers by changing the hormonal and cellular micro-environment in which the cancer cells strive to multiply (chapters 2 and 6). A logical consequence of this view is that while some cancer cells may die in the new surroundings, others that can tolerate the new, changed environment will survive; thus the tumours, after a period of remission, may begin to grow again. This is of course what happens in many cases in patients treated with chemotherapy—there is a selection of cells resistant to the drug. As with chemotherapy, so with psychotherapy: patients may need to "keep on the move," continuing to evolve and grow psychologically and spiritually, to outpace or outwit their evolving cancer cell populations! While some people may reach a point where they are sufficiently "healed" to shake off their disease, others, either because they reach a plateau in their healing efforts or because they have more resistant and aggressive cancers, may simply buy themselves some time, of the order of a year or two. This is what we think we observe in our program participants. However, data are much too scant to be sure, and a great deal of painstaking research is needed to test ideas such as these.

Subjects for Research

Because the benefits of psychological work are not yet clear enough to induce most people to become involved in it, we need to focus first on that minority of patients who are willing and able to make an effort. Relevant change can be achieved through a stepwise program like the one I described in chapter 5, in which those individuals who are most keen on self-healing identify themselves. These people will teach us what is possible. Armed with that knowledge, we will have a better chance of convincing more skeptical individuals that psychological and spiritual self-help are worth attempting. The methods will also need to be tailored to fit populations differing in educational and cultural backgrounds.

The Therapy

Self-healing is a *learned* process; thus the first requirement for work of this kind is that it provide education as well as support. Many community centres for cancer patients miss this point, and offer only the supportive function. Incorporating a guiding structure for the patient's growth is essential, I believe, because without that, relatively few will mount a truly constructive and potentially healing response. This statement is based on decades of watching people struggle to understand how to help themselves. Like education in other areas, self-healing is progressive: one learns simple things first, like relaxation and keeping the mind relatively quiet, then builds on them with more sophisticated ideas. The stepwise program I outlined in chapter 5 is one way of providing a progressive, educational structure, one that allows participants to determine for themselves how much of the work they will do.

As in most areas of human endeavour, it is only sensible to seek help from more experienced people. These teacher/therapists need to have training in both the process of psychological therapy for the physically ill, and experience in the techniques they teach. As teachers, we must practise what we preach. This requirement can deter some health care professionals who are accustomed to being less personally involved with their ministrations. Training others in self-help is in many ways analogous to teaching a foreign language, or a musical instrument, where it is taken for granted that the teacher will be proficient.

The patients themselves will generally be psychologically normal (apart from some anxiety or depression, caused by their disease), so there is no need for the exclusive focus on psychopathology that is common in counselling—instead, we can follow LeShan's advice and concentrate on "what would be right for the person," an approach validated by our research results. The widely varying needs and abilities of different individuals must be respected; some may need to spend longer at different "levels" of a therapy program, while others (particularly any with long-standing psychopathology) may need supplementary one-to-one therapy.

Professionally led groups, rather than individual (one-to-one) meetings, are particularly useful, both for reasons of economy and because the interaction and support between peers is an important part of the healing. In a well-led group with people who are at ease with one another, there is some healing at work at a sub-verbal level that I don't pretend to understand, but have often felt; perhaps it is a form of loving connection, like that operating in the distant prayer experiments cited above. Currently, many people with cancer don't want to join a therapeutic group; research is needed to clarify the reasons for this reluctance, but from my observation I think that most people are unfamiliar with the group process, and afraid of what they might be asked to expose about themselves. Stoical attitudes are common ("I should handle this by myself"), and seeking psychological help is sometimes taken as indicating mental illness or weakness in the recipient. These anxieties and misconceptions usually vanish rapidly with experience, and are replaced by warm appreciation for the other group members. Initial reluctance to take part can be minimized if the educational and stress reduction aims are emphasized (for example, we call our first-level group "Coping with Cancer Stress").

The essence of our approach is to provide a structured, stepwise educational program including a variety of techniques, presented in a graded fashion, and relying on the patient taking considerable initiative. People with cancer who want more information on the specific material we cover will find it in my earlier books. It is likely that there are many other routes to physical healing, just as there are many kinds of psychotherapy that lead to mental healing, but claims do need to be documented. We can be guided by our growing knowledge of the main psychological qualities accompanying healing, which I've tentatively described as authenticity, autonomy, and acceptance; methods should logically be used that help people attain these states of mind. Whatever approach is adopted needs to bring about changes relatively quickly, if the cancer is serious; thus intensity is important. We ask participants to do a lot of introspective work at home and write about it, submitting copies for our comments, and this greatly accelerates the learning. Lengthy retreats in places providing suitable guidance are another way of increasing intensity. There is an advantage to offering a smorgasbord of methods, since it allows people to choose which techniques help them most. And the process must be flexible enough to support the varied ways in which people learn and operate.

OVERALL CONCLUSIONS: CAN THE MIND "HEAL" CANCER?

Can the mind heal cancer? We discussed, in chapter 1, the need to clarify what we mean by this question. There is no doubt that much of the mental suffering caused by cancer can be alleviated by deliberate mental action on the part of the suffering person—something as simple as practising a relaxation technique can relieve anxiety and pain. But what the person asking this question usually means is, "Can a person with cancer make changes within her mind that lead to better conditions in the body for healing an existing cancer?" meaning slowing or even reversing the growth of tumours. This is the main topic addressed in this book. It is one that has stirred a lot of New Age passion and much adverse reaction from many medical authorities. My attempt here has been to put forward a synthesis of new evidence and older theory and clinical observation that I think shows there are real possibilities for a degree of healing through the mind, although the process is by no means as simple as some popular accounts would claim.

We saw that there is already a lot of evidence for mind affecting disease, and that this may be understood in terms of mental "software" influencing body "hardware." Some of the mechanisms by which this might happen are known; for example, we have a fair understanding of the effects of psychological stress on hormone production and subsequently on the functions of the immune system (chapter 2). More generally, it seems reasonable to propose that diminishing a habit of constant defensiveness will allow those systems of the body that are responsible for maintaining health to operate more effectively. Then we reviewed the descriptive studies on remarkable survivors, which have generated a rather consistent picture of the qualities associated with healing, in spite of the weakness of that approach. By contrast, more orthodox studies in modern psycho-oncology have failed to tell us much so far, and I explain why: basically, the methods used have not been very appropriate to the questions asked. The core of the book was devoted to a new approach, outlined in chapters 5 and 6, its essence being the case-by-case documentation of what people with serious cancers think and do over a prolonged period, then relating these psychological data to the subsequent duration of survival. This demonstrated a highly significant relationship between degree of involvement in psychological and spiritual self-help methods, and survival. We also interviewed a number of long survivors, under relatively controlled conditions, obtaining results very similar to the more informal "remarkable survivor" studies published earlier.

Putting all of this together with a theory first advanced some 20 years ago by scientist Lydia Temoshok, and seminal clinical observations by the psycho-oncology pioneer Lawrence LeShan, we arrive at the following synthesis: cancer seems to progress more rapidly in people who adopt a placatory, self-denying style of thinking and acting (Temoshok's data, discussed in chapter 4). Those individuals who overcome a serious cancer show a precise reversal of this pattern, claiming instead the right to live in ways that they decide are fulfilling for them. There is a mirrored symmetry here between the mental characteristics that may promote cancer and those that may oppose it, and there is good agreement about the latter between our own investigations and those of other authors. Thus although no one piece of evidence is conclusive by itself, these strands converge. What is more, they add up to a hypothesis that makes good sense: simply put, relieve longstanding strain on your mind, and it will free up the body to oppose disease more effectively.

A FINAL WORD TO PEOPLE WITH CANCER

If you have read through this short text, you will see that there is considerable evidence for a potential healing effect of your state of mind on cancer, in a way that can be rationally explained. You will meet people who make much grander claims, who perhaps have magical remedies on offer. In evaluating them, you may wish to ask three questions:

- Is there evidence for the effectiveness of these remedies or procedures?
- Is there a consensus that they work (among people who have studied them)?
- Is there some way of understanding how they might work—do they make sense?

You will find, unfortunately, that most of the "alternative remedies" fail all three tests, as I discuss further in *The Healing Journey*. The situation is quite different when we consider the healing impact of directed mental change—as you have seen, we can answer a qualified "yes" to all three questions. You may encounter opposition to this assertion from orthodox health care professionals, in which case it is fair to ask them what study they have made of the effects of mind on disease. Give them this book: I don't believe that any nurse, doctor, social worker, or other trained health professional could find it unreasonable—the worst verdict they might return is "insufficient evidence to convince me."

If you have cancer, or some other serious health condition, should you try to do this mental healing work? Obviously I think so. Try to find an experienced guide; if there is nobody available who works with clients who have your kind of medical condition, then consider attending a school of "personal growth" or spirituality that aims to help people escape from the limitations of habitual thinking. A lot of books on psychological change are available these days. Look around for a psychotherapist with an interest in this kind of work. Avoid people charging very high prices or making dogmatic claims. You may have to put together your own "program"—to construct a patch-work quilt, rather than hoping to find a ready-made coverall.

In the end, it is an individual decision how to respond to life-threatening illness. We can choose to be active or passive. If we are afraid to try and "fail," then we may never get started. Consider other areas of your life, where you may have been willing to attempt some-thing challenging, even when success was far from assured. Self-healing is not different in this respect. There is no need for blam-ing oneself if we try to assist our healing, yet the disease continues to progress: we know very little about the process as yet, and many cancers may be resistant to even the greatest efforts, either medical or mental. What we can be sure of is that our experience of cancer or other life-threatening disease will be very different if we respond actively, rather than remaining a passive victim of events. Our quality of life, our self-respect, will be enhanced. We may also come to un-derstand that physical well-being is not necessarily the primary aim of life, and we may gain, from spiritual searching, an awareness that we are much more than just our bodies or our minds.

REFERENCES

1. Cunningham, A. J. (2002). *Bringing spirituality into your healing journey.* Toronto: Key Porter.

2. Happold, H. C. (1970). *Mysticism: A study and an anthology* (Rev. ed.). London: Penguin, 20.

3. Aldridge, D. (1993). Is there evidence for spiritual healing? *Advances, 9*(4), 4–21.
   Levin, J. S. (1993). Esoteric vs. exoteric explanations for findings linking spirituality and health. *Advances, 9*(4), 54–56.
   Powell, L. H., Shahabi, L., & Thoresen, C. E. (2003). Religion and spirituality: Linkages to physical health. *American Psychologist, 58*(1), 36–52.
   Seeman, T. E., Dubin, L. F., & Seeman, J. (2003). Religiosity/spirituality and health: A critical review of the evidence for biological pathways. *American Psychologist, 58*(1), 53–63.
   Thoresen, C. E., & Harris, A. H. S. (2002). Spirituality and health: What's the evidence and what's needed? *Annals of Behavioral Medicine, 24*(1), 3–13.

4. Jahn, R. G., & Dunne, B. J. (1987). *Margins of reality: The role of consciousness in the physical world.* New York: Harcourt Brace Jovanovich.

5. Larry Dossey is the physician who has perhaps done most to champion what he calls "non-local healing," in a series of books and in his excellent editorials for the new scientific journal *Alternative Therapies.*
   Some of Dr. Dossey's many books:
   Dossey, L. (1982). *Space, time and medicine.* Boston: Shambhala.
   Dossey, L. (1989). *Recovering the soul: A scientific and spiritual search.* New York: Bantam.
   Dossey, L. (1999). *Reinventing medicine: Beyond mind–body to a new era of healing.* San Francisco: Harper.